I0696929

Copyright © 2023 Izabela Zieba

All rights reserved.

ISBN: 9798861662383

DEAR TEA LOVERS,

Whether it's an herbal tea or an earl grey with orange peels, I dedicate this lovely book to all tea lovers out there. I hope you'll find your favorite recipe right here. Enjoy!

Nowadays, everybody is talking about healthier life choices. But working 8am-5pm, being a mom and a housewife doesn't really leave you much time to even think about healthier life choices, neither for you nor for your family. I have decided that I must start somewhere. As a complete tea lover, I decided that I will start with… tea.

I have grown up on a small farm and I always knew that all weeds in our garden are really herbs in disguise. My grandma was always making some "green potions" in a big jug. She used to put different weeds from the field outside our house and pour boiling water over it. I'll be honest with you: at the time it looked disgusting.

One day I thought, why not try my grandma "recipe" …

Herbs, particularly when used in tea, offer a wide range of positive properties that can benefit our overall health and well-being. These properties have been appreciated for centuries, and herbal teas are enjoyed worldwide for their natural healing and soothing effects. Here are some of the positive properties of herbs, especially when used in tea:

1. Calming and Relaxing:

- Many herbs, such as chamomile, lavender, and lemon balm, have calming and relaxing properties. They can help reduce stress, anxiety, and promote a sense of calm.

2. Digestive Support:

- Peppermint, ginger, and fennel are herbs commonly used to aid digestion. They can help relieve symptoms of indigestion, bloating, and nausea.

3. Immune Boosting:

- Herbs like echinacea, elderberry, and astragalus are known for their immune-boosting properties. They can help strengthen the body's defenses against infections.

4. Anti-Inflammatory:

- Turmeric and ginger are well-known for their anti-inflammatory properties. They may help reduce inflammation and ease discomfort associated with conditions like arthritis.

5. Antioxidant-Rich:

- Many herbs, such as green tea, rosehip, and hibiscus, are rich in antioxidants. These compounds help protect cells from oxidative stress and reduce the risk of chronic diseases.

6. Sleep Aid:

- Herbs like valerian, chamomile, and passionflower can promote relaxation and improve sleep quality. They are often used as natural remedies for insomnia.

7. Pain Relief:

- Willow bark, like aspirin, has been used historically for pain relief. It may help alleviate headaches, muscle aches, and mild pain.

8. Respiratory Support:

- Herbs like eucalyptus, thyme, and liquorice root can support respiratory health. They may help alleviate symptoms of colds, coughs, and congestion.

9. Hormonal Balance:

- Herbs like red clover and black cohosh are used to support hormonal balance in women, particularly during menopause.

10. Skin Health: - Calendula (commonly called pot marigold), lavender, and nettle are herbs known for their potential benefits for skin health. They can soothe irritations, reduce inflammation, and promote healing.

11. Detoxification: - Dandelion root and milk thistle are commonly used for their potential detoxifying properties. They may support liver health and aid in the elimination of toxins.

12. Weight Management: - Green tea, in particular, is often associated with weight management due to its potential to boost metabolism and aid in fat oxidation.

13. Hydration: - Herbal teas are a great way to stay hydrated, which is essential for overall health. Unlike caffeinated beverages, herbal teas are typically caffeine-free.

14. Customizable: - Herbal teas offer a wide variety of flavours and properties, allowing individuals to choose the herbs that suit their specific needs and preferences.

15. Natural and Safe: - Herbal teas are a natural and safe way to promote health and wellness. They are often free of artificial additives and preservatives.

It's important to note that the effectiveness of herbal teas can vary among individuals, and not all herbs are suitable for everyone. If you have specific health concerns or are pregnant, it's advisable to consult with a healthcare professional or herbalist before using herbal teas for medicinal purposes. Nonetheless, incorporating herbal teas into your daily routine can be a soothing and enjoyable way to support your health and promote overall well-being.

Let's start with a simple one: nettle tea.

Nettle tea is an herbal infusion made from the leaves of the stinging nettle plant (Urtica dioica). It's known for its earthy and slightly grassy flavour and is often enjoyed for its potential health benefits, including its high nutrient content and anti-inflammatory properties. Here's a simple recipe for making nettle tea.

NETTLE TEA RECIPE

Ingredients:

- 1 to 2 teaspoons of dried nettle leaves (or 1 nettle tea bag)
- 1 cup of boiling water
- Optional additions: honey, lemon, or other herbs for flavour

Instructions:

- **Prepare the Nettle Leaves:**
    - If you're using fresh nettle leaves, be cautious as they can sting. Wear gloves or use tongs to handle them until they're dried or steeped in hot water, which neutralizes the stinging hairs. If you're using dried nettle leaves or a tea bag, you can skip this step.
- **Boil Water:**
    - Boil water in a kettle or on the stovetop. You'll need about one cup (8 ounces) of boiling water for each serving of nettle tea.
- **Place Nettle Leaves in a Cup:**
    - If using loose-leaf dried nettle, place 1 to 2 teaspoons of dried nettle leaves into a teacup or teapot. If you have a nettle tea bag, you can place it directly into the cup.
- **Pour Boiling Water:**
    - Carefully pour the boiling water over the nettle leaves or tea bag. Ensure the leaves or tea bag are fully submerged.
- **Steep:**
    - Allow the nettle leaves to steep in the hot water for about 5-7 minutes. You can adjust the steeping time to

> your taste, but be cautious not to over-steep, as nettle tea can become quite strong and slightly bitter if left too long.

- **Remove the Leaves or Tea Bag:**
    - After steeping, remove the nettle leaves or tea bag from the cup. You can use a tea strainer or simply lift out the tea bag.
- **Optional Additions:**
    - If desired, you can sweeten your nettle tea with honey or add a squeeze of lemon for flavour. Nettle tea has an earthy taste, and these additions can complement its flavour.
- **Enjoy:**
    - Your nettle tea is now ready to enjoy. Sip it while it's still warm.

Note: Nettle tea is generally safe for most people, but if you have allergies or are pregnant, it's best to consult with a healthcare professional before consuming it regularly. Additionally, if you plan to forage for fresh nettle leaves, make sure you can positively identify the plant and handle it with care to avoid stings. **Always wash fresh nettle leaves thoroughly before using them in tea.**

It was so simple! I used fresh nettle, and I was so proud of myself! I felt healthier already.

Fresh nettles, specifically the leaves and young shoots of the stinging nettle plant (Urtica dioica), are known for their potential health benefits and various properties. Here are some of the key properties and characteristics of fresh nettles:

1. Nutrient-Rich:

- Fresh nettles are highly nutritious and packed with vitamins and minerals. They are an excellent source of vitamin C, vitamin K, vitamin A, and several B vitamins. They also contain minerals such as iron, calcium, magnesium, and potassium.

2. Anti-Inflammatory:

- Nettles have anti-inflammatory properties and may help reduce inflammation in the body. They are often used to alleviate symptoms of inflammatory conditions such as arthritis.

3. Allergy Relief:

- Contrary to their stinging reputation, consuming fresh nettle leaves in various forms, such as tea or soup, is believed by some to help relieve symptoms of seasonal allergies. Some people use nettle supplements to alleviate hay fever.

4. Diuretic Effect:

- Fresh nettles have diuretic properties, which means they can increase urine production. This can help with conditions involving fluid retention and may support kidney health.

5. Antioxidant Properties:

- Nettles contain antioxidants, such as flavonoids and carotenoids, which help combat oxidative stress and protect cells from damage caused by free radicals.

6. Potential for Lowering Blood Pressure:

- Some studies suggest that nettle extracts may help lower blood pressure, although more research is needed in this area.

7. Digestive Health:

- Nettles have been used traditionally to support digestive health. They may help with indigestion and improve overall gut function.

8. Hair and Skin Care:

- Nettles are sometimes used in hair and skincare products for their potential benefits. Nettle extracts may promote hair growth and alleviate dandruff. Additionally, they may have anti-inflammatory effects on the skin.

9. Culinary Uses:

- Young, tender nettle leaves can be harvested and cooked in a similar way to spinach or used in various culinary dishes. They are often added to soups, stews, and omelets. Nettle tea made from fresh leaves is also popular.

10. Environmental Benefits: - Nettles play a role in ecosystems by providing habitat and food for various insects and wildlife. They are also valued in permaculture and organic gardening for their nutrient-rich compost.

11. Sustainable Foraging: - Nettles are easily found in many regions and can be sustainably foraged. When harvesting fresh nettles, it's essential to use gloves to avoid the stinging hairs on the leaves.

12. Potential for Traditional Medicine: - Nettles have a long history of use in traditional herbal medicine for a variety of ailments, including joint pain, urinary tract issues, and skin conditions.

While fresh nettles offer several potential health benefits, it's essential to use them with care. The stinging hairs on the leaves can cause skin irritation, so it's recommended to wear gloves when handling fresh nettles. Additionally, consult with a healthcare professional before using nettles for medicinal purposes, especially if you have specific health conditions or are taking medications.

POT MARIGOLD, LAVENDER AND NETTLE TEA

To help with your skin health you can prepare this easy to make calendula (pot marigold), lavender and nettle tea.

Calendula, lavender, and nettle tea is a delightful herbal blend that combines the soothing and aromatic qualities of these herbs. Here's a simple recipe to make this herbal tea:

Ingredients:

- 1 tablespoon dried calendula flowers
- 1 tablespoon dried lavender flowers
- 1 tablespoon dried nettle leaves
- 2 cups of boiling water
- Honey or lemon (optional, for flavour)
- Fresh lavender sprig or calendula petals (optional, for garnish)

Instructions:

- **Prepare the Herbs:**
  - Measure out 1 tablespoon each of dried calendula flowers, dried lavender flowers, and dried nettle leaves. You can adjust the quantities to suit your taste.
- **Boil Water:**
  - Bring 2 cups (16 ounces) of water to a rolling boil in a kettle or on the stovetop.
- **Combine the Herbs:**
  - In a teapot or heatproof container, combine the dried calendula flowers, dried lavender flowers, and dried nettle leaves.
- **Pour Boiling Water:**
  - Carefully pour the boiling water over the dried herbs in the teapot or container.
- **Steep:**
  - Cover the teapot or container and let the herbs steep in the hot water for about 5-7 minutes. This allows the flavours and properties of the herbs to infuse into the

> water. You can adjust the steeping time to your taste, but avoid over-steeping, as it can make the tea overly strong.

- **Strain (Optional):**
    - If you prefer not to have herbs in your tea, strain the tea as you pour it into your cup using a fine-mesh strainer.
- **Optional Additions:**
    - If desired, sweeten your tea with honey or add a squeeze of lemon for extra flavour. Calendula, lavender, and nettle tea have pleasant and soothing flavours, and these additions can enhance the overall experience.
- **Garnish (Optional):**
    - For an extra touch of elegance, you can garnish your tea with a fresh lavender sprig or a few calendula petals.
- **Serve:**
    - Your calendula, lavender, and nettle tea is now ready to enjoy. Sip it while it's still warm and savour the soothing and aromatic qualities of this herbal blend.

This herbal tea is known for its calming and relaxing properties, making it an excellent choice for winding down after a long day or enjoying a moment of tranquility. Additionally, the combination of these herbs offers potential benefits for skin health, relaxation, and overall well-being.

Calendula

Calendula, commonly known as pot marigold (Calendula officinalis), is a versatile herb that offers a wide range of properties and potential health benefits. It has been used for centuries in traditional medicine, culinary applications, and skincare products. Here are some of the notable properties and characteristics of calendula:

1. Anti-Inflammatory:

- Calendula possesses anti-inflammatory properties and may help reduce inflammation and related discomfort when applied topically or consumed as an herbal remedy.

2. Skin Health:

- Calendula is well-known for its benefits to the skin. It is used in creams, ointments, and salves to soothe and heal various skin conditions, including minor burns, cuts, rashes, and insect bites.

3. Wound Healing:

- Calendula promotes wound healing by stimulating tissue regeneration. It can be used to speed up the recovery of minor wounds and abrasions.

4. Antioxidant Content:

- Calendula is rich in antioxidants, which help protect cells from oxidative stress and free radical damage. Antioxidants may have various health benefits, including supporting overall wellness.

5. Immune Support:

- Calendula has immune-boosting properties and may help strengthen the body's defenses against infections and illnesses.

6. Anti-Microbial:

- Calendula exhibits antimicrobial properties and can be used to reduce the risk of infection when applied to minor wounds or skin irritations.

7. Calming and Relaxing:

- Calendula has a soothing and calming effect when used in teas or aromatherapy. It can help reduce stress and anxiety.

8. Digestive Aid:

- Calendula tea may support digestion and alleviate symptoms of indigestion, gas, and bloating.

9. Menstrual Health:

- Calendula is sometimes used to relieve menstrual cramps and discomfort when consumed as a tea.

10. Anti-Fungal: - Calendula may help combat fungal infections when used topically or as part of a skin care regimen.

11. Gastrointestinal Health: - Calendula tea may help soothe inflammation in the gastrointestinal tract and alleviate symptoms of conditions like gastritis.

12. Culinary Uses: - Calendula petals are edible and can be used as a colourful garnish in salads, soups, and other dishes. They have a slightly peppery flavour.

13. Eye Health: - Calendula tea can be used as an eyewash to relieve eye irritations and reduce inflammation.

14. Anti-Spasmodic: - Calendula tea may help reduce muscle spasms and cramps when consumed.

15. Hair Care: - Calendula-infused oils and shampoos are used to promote healthy hair and soothe scalp conditions.

16. Aromatherapy: - Calendula essential oil, extracted from the flowers, is used in aromatherapy for its calming and skin-soothing properties.

Calendula can be consumed as a tea, applied topically as an ointment or cream, or used in various forms in skincare products. It is generally considered safe for most people when used as directed. However, if you have specific allergies or sensitivities, it's advisable to perform a patch test or consult with a healthcare professional before using calendula products. Additionally, pregnant or nursing individuals should consult with a healthcare provider before using calendula in significant amounts.

Lavender

Lavender (Lavandula spp.) is a fragrant herb known for its distinctive aroma and a wide range of properties that have made it popular in various cultural and medicinal practices. Lavender possesses numerous positive properties and potential health benefits, making it one of the most versatile and beloved herbs. Here are some of the notable properties and characteristics of lavender:

1. Relaxing and Calming:

- Lavender is perhaps best known for its calming and relaxing properties. The scent of lavender has been shown to reduce stress, anxiety, and promote a sense of calm and well-being.

2. Aromatherapy:

- Lavender essential oil is commonly used in aromatherapy to alleviate stress, improve sleep quality, and promote relaxation. It can be diffused, added to bathwater, or used in massage oils.

3. Sleep Aid:

- Lavender is used to improve sleep quality and treat insomnia. Placing dried lavender sachets under your pillow or using lavender essential oil in a diffuser can help you sleep more soundly.

4. Analgesic (Pain-Relieving):

- Lavender essential oil, when applied topically, may help relieve minor aches and pains. It can be used in massage oils or added to bathwater for a relaxing soak.

5. Anti-Inflammatory:

- Lavender possesses anti-inflammatory properties and may help reduce inflammation and related discomfort when applied topically or consumed as a tea.

6. Skin Health:

- Lavender is used to soothe and heal various skin conditions, including minor burns, cuts, insect bites, and acne. It has antiseptic and antimicrobial properties.

7. Wound Healing:

- Lavender promotes wound healing and tissue regeneration. It can be applied to minor wounds and abrasions to speed up the healing process.

8. Antioxidant Content:

- Lavender contains antioxidants, which help protect cells from oxidative stress and free radical damage. Antioxidants have various health benefits.

9. Immune Support:

- Lavender has immune-boosting properties and may help strengthen the body's defenses against infections and illnesses.

10. Respiratory Health: - Lavender-infused steam inhalation or tea can help relieve respiratory discomfort, such as coughs, colds, and congestion.

11. Digestive Aid: - Lavender tea is sometimes used to support digestion, alleviate symptoms of indigestion, gas, and bloating.

12. Hair Care: - Lavender-infused hair products can promote healthy hair and soothe scalp conditions like dandruff.

13. Culinary Uses: - Lavender flowers are edible and can be used in culinary applications, including baking, teas, and flavouring desserts and beverages.

14. Headache Relief: - Lavender essential oil or lavender-infused balms are sometimes used to relieve tension headaches and migraines when applied to the temples and forehead.

15. Natural Perfume: - Lavender's pleasant fragrance makes it a popular natural perfume and addition to sachets and potpourri.

16. Antiseptic: - Lavender has antiseptic properties, which can help prevent infections when applied to minor wounds and cuts.

Lavender can be used in various forms, including as an essential oil, dried flowers, teas, and topical products. It is generally considered safe for most people when used as directed. However, if you have specific allergies or sensitivities, it's advisable to perform a patch test or consult with a healthcare professional before using lavender products. Lavender's calming and healing properties have made it a beloved herb in many cultures and a staple in herbal medicine and aromatherapy.

Another simple one is dandelion tea.

DANDELION TEA

Dandelion tea is a popular herbal infusion made from the dried leaves and roots of the dandelion plant (Taraxacum officinale). It is known for its potential health benefits and its slightly bitter and earthy flavour. Here's a simple recipe for making dandelion tea from dried dandelion leaves:

Ingredients:

- 1 to 2 teaspoons of dried dandelion leaves (or dandelion tea bags)
- 1 cup of boiling water
- Optional additions: honey, lemon, or other herbs for flavour

Instructions:

- **Prepare the Dandelion Leaves:**
    - If you're using dried dandelion leaves, measure out 1 to 2 teaspoons per cup of tea. You can adjust the amount to your taste, but be cautious not to use too many leaves, as dandelion tea can become quite bitter when steeped for an extended period.
- **Boil Water:**
    - Boil water in a kettle or on the stovetop. You'll need about one cup (8 ounces) of boiling water for each serving of dandelion tea.
- **Place Dandelion Leaves in a Cup:**
    - If using loose-leaf dried dandelion leaves, place them into a teacup or teapot. If you have dandelion tea bags, you can place one tea bag directly into the cup.
- **Pour Boiling Water:**
    - Carefully pour the boiling water over the dandelion leaves or tea bag. Make sure the leaves or tea bag are fully submerged.
- **Steep:**
    - Allow the dandelion leaves to steep in the hot water for about 5-7 minutes. Adjust the steeping time to your taste, but avoid over-steeping, as it can make the tea overly bitter.
- **Remove the Leaves or Tea Bag:**
    - After steeping, remove the dandelion leaves or tea bag from the cup. You can use a tea strainer or simply lift out the tea bag.
- **Optional Additions:**
    - If desired, you can sweeten your dandelion tea with honey or add a squeeze of lemon for flavour. Dandelion tea has an earthy taste, and these additions can complement its flavour.
- **Enjoy:**
    - Your dandelion tea is ready to enjoy. Sip it while it's still warm.

Note: Dandelion tea is generally safe for most people, but if you have allergies or are pregnant, it's best to consult with a healthcare professional before consuming it regularly. Dandelion tea is known for its potential diuretic properties, so consider this if you're sensitive to diuretics or have a medical condition that may be affected by increased urine output. Additionally, when foraging for fresh dandelion leaves, make sure you can positively identify the plant and harvest from areas free of pesticides and contaminants. Always wash fresh dandelion leaves thoroughly before using them in tea.

Dried dandelion, typically made from the leaves and roots of the dandelion plant (Taraxacum officinale), is used for a variety of purposes, including as a herbal remedy and culinary ingredient. Here are some of the key properties and characteristics of dried dandelion:

1. Nutrient-Rich:

- Dried dandelion leaves and roots are rich in essential nutrients. They are a good source of vitamins and minerals, including vitamin A, vitamin C, vitamin K, vitamin E, iron, calcium, potassium, and magnesium.

2. Digestive Health:

- Dandelion has a long history of use in traditional herbal medicine for its digestive properties. It is believed to stimulate the production of digestive juices, promote healthy digestion, and alleviate symptoms of indigestion and bloating.

3. Diuretic Effect:

- Dandelion is known for its diuretic properties, which means it can increase urine production. This can help with conditions involving fluid retention and may support kidney and urinary tract health.

4. Liver Health:

- Dandelion has been used to support liver health and detoxification processes. It is believed to promote the flow of bile, which aids in the digestion of fats and the elimination of toxins.

5. Antioxidant Properties:

- Dandelion contains antioxidants, including flavonoids, which help combat oxidative stress and protect cells from damage caused by free radicals.

6. Potential Anti-Inflammatory Effects:

- Some studies suggest that dandelion may have anti-inflammatory properties, which can be beneficial for conditions involving inflammation and pain.

7. Potential Blood Sugar Regulation:

- There is some evidence to suggest that dandelion may help regulate blood sugar levels and improve insulin sensitivity, which could be beneficial for individuals with diabetes or those at risk of developing it.

8. Weight Management:

- Dandelion leaves are low in calories and can be included in a weight management plan to provide bulk and reduce calorie intake.

9. Skin Health:

- Dandelion extracts are sometimes used in skincare products for their potential to soothe skin irritations and promote healthy skin. They may also help reduce the appearance of blemishes and dark spots.

10. Culinary Uses: - Dandelion leaves and roots can be dried and ground into a powder or used fresh in culinary dishes. Dried dandelion leaves can be used in teas, soups, salads, and as a flavouring for baked goods.

11. Traditional Medicine: - Dandelion has a history of use in traditional medicine systems, including Traditional Chinese Medicine (TCM) and traditional European herbalism, for a wide range of health concerns.

12. Potential Allergy Relief: - Some people use dandelion supplements or tea to alleviate allergy symptoms, such as runny nose and itchy eyes, although scientific evidence is limited.

13. Environmental Benefits: - Dandelions are hardy plants and are often seen as valuable in permaculture and organic gardening practices. They can attract pollinators and improve soil health.

14. Sustainable Foraging: - Dandelions are easily found in many regions and can be sustainably foraged for culinary and medicinal purposes. When foraging for fresh dandelion leaves and roots, make sure you can positively identify the plant and harvest from areas free of pesticides and contaminants.

As with any herbal remedy, it's important to consult with a healthcare professional before using dried dandelion for therapeutic purposes, especially if you have specific medical conditions or are taking medications. Additionally, ensure that you are sourcing dried dandelion from reputable sources to guarantee quality and purity.

DANDELION ROOT AND MILK THISTLE TEA

Dandelion root and milk thistle are two herbs known for their potential benefits in supporting liver health and digestion. Combining them in a tea or infusion can create a soothing and beneficial beverage. Here's a simple recipe for a dandelion root and milk thistle tea:

Ingredients:

- 1 tablespoon dried dandelion root
- 1 tablespoon dried milk thistle seeds
- 2 cups of water
- Honey or lemon (optional, for flavour)

Instructions:

- **Prepare the Herbs:**
    - Measure out 1 tablespoon each of dried dandelion root and dried milk thistle seeds. You can adjust the quantities to your taste.
- **Boil Water:**
    - Bring 2 cups (16 ounces) of water to a rolling boil in a kettle or on the stovetop.
- **Combine the Herbs:**
    - In a teapot or heatproof container, combine the dried dandelion root and dried milk thistle seeds.
- **Pour Boiling Water:**
    - Carefully pour the boiling water over the dried herbs in the teapot or container.
- **Steep:**
    - Cover the teapot or container and let the herbs steep in the hot water for about 10-15 minutes. This allows the flavours and properties of the herbs to infuse into the water. You can adjust the steeping time to your taste, but avoid over-steeping, as it can make the tea overly strong.
- **Strain (Optional):**
    - If you prefer not to have herbs in your tea, strain the tea as you pour it into your cup using a fine-mesh strainer.
- **Optional Additions:**
    - If desired, sweeten your tea with honey or add a squeeze of lemon for extra flavour. Dandelion root and milk thistle tea have a slightly earthy and bitter taste, and these additions can make it more palatable.
- **Serve:**
    - Your dandelion root and milk thistle tea is now ready to enjoy. Sip it while it's still warm and savour the potential

benefits of this herbal blend for liver health and digestion.

This herbal tea is known for its potential benefits in supporting liver detoxification and promoting healthy digestion. Both dandelion root and milk thistle are believed to have properties that support the liver's natural functions and help alleviate digestive discomfort. Additionally, this tea may have mild diuretic properties, so be mindful of fluid intake when consuming it. As with any herbal remedy, it's advisable to consult with a healthcare professional if you have specific health concerns or are taking medications, as herbs can interact with certain medications.

Milk thistle (Silybum marianum) is a flowering plant known for its various medicinal properties, particularly its benefits for liver health. The active ingredient in milk thistle is a group of compounds called silymarin. Here are some of the key properties and potential health benefits of milk thistle:

1. Liver Protection: Milk thistle is most famous for its hepatoprotective (liverprotecting) properties. Silymarin, the primary component, has antioxidant and anti-inflammatory effects that can help protect liver cells from damage caused by toxins, such as alcohol, pollution, and certain medications.

2. Detoxification: Milk thistle may support the liver in detoxifying the body by increasing the production of enzymes involved in the detoxification process. This can assist in the removal of harmful substances from the body.

3. Liver Regeneration: Silymarin has been shown in some studies to stimulate the regeneration of liver tissue. This can be beneficial for people with liver diseases like cirrhosis or hepatitis.

4. Antioxidant Properties: Silymarin acts as a powerful antioxidant, helping to neutralize harmful free radicals in the body. This antioxidant activity can have positive effects on overall health, as oxidative stress is linked to various chronic diseases.

5. Anti-Inflammatory Effects: Milk thistle has anti-inflammatory properties that can benefit not only the liver but also other parts of the body. Chronic inflammation is associated with a range of health issues, and milk thistle's anti-inflammatory effects may help mitigate some of these problems.

6. Cholesterol Management: Some research suggests that milk thistle may help lower LDL (bad) cholesterol levels in the blood. This can contribute to better cardiovascular health.

7. Diabetes Management: There is evidence to suggest that milk thistle may have a role in helping regulate blood sugar levels. It may improve insulin sensitivity and reduce blood sugar spikes.

8. Gallbladder Health: Milk thistle may be used to promote gallbladder health and reduce the risk of gallstones.

9. Skin Health: Some topical preparations containing milk thistle extracts are used for various skin conditions, such as acne and psoriasis, due to its anti-inflammatory and antioxidant properties. It's important to note that while milk thistle has numerous potential benefits, it should be used with caution, and it's advisable to consult with a healthcare professional before using it as a supplement, especially if you have underlying health conditions or are taking medications. Additionally, the quality and dosage of milk thistle supplements can vary, so it's essential to choose reputable products if you decide to incorporate it into your health regimen.

DAISY TEA

Daisy tea, often made from dried daisy flowers, is a soothing and mildly floral herbal infusion. It's known for its potential calming properties and pleasant taste. Here's a simple recipe for you:

Ingredients:

- 1 to 2 teaspoons of dried daisy flowers (or daisy tea bags)
- 1 cup of boiling water
- Optional additions: honey or a slice of lemon for flavour

Instructions:

- **Prepare the Daisy Flowers:**
  - If you're using dried daisy flowers, measure out 1 to 2 teaspoons per cup of tea. You can adjust the amount to your taste, but be cautious not to use too many flowers, as daisy tea can become overly floral if steeped for too long.
- **Boil Water:**
  - Boil water in a kettle or on the stovetop. You'll need about one cup (8 ounces) of boiling water for each serving of daisy tea.
- **Place Daisy Flowers in a Cup:**
  - If using loose-leaf dried daisy flowers, place them into a teacup or teapot. If you have daisy tea bags, you can place one tea bag directly into the cup.
- **Pour Boiling Water:**
  - Carefully pour the boiling water over the daisy flowers or tea bag. Ensure the flowers or tea bag are fully submerged.
- **Steep:**
  - Allow the daisy flowers to steep in the hot water for about 5-7 minutes. Adjust the steeping time to your taste, but avoid over-steeping, as it can make the tea too floral.
- **Remove the Flowers or Tea Bag:**
  - After steeping, remove the daisy flowers or tea bag from the cup. You can use a tea strainer or simply lift out the tea bag.
- **Optional Additions:**
  - If desired, you can sweeten your daisy tea with honey or add a slice of lemon for a hint of citrus flavour. Daisy tea has a delicate taste, and these additions can enhance its overall profile.
- **Enjoy:**
  - Your daisy tea is now ready to enjoy. Sip it while it's still warm.

Note: Daisy tea is generally considered safe for most people. However, it's advisable to consult with a healthcare professional before consuming it regularly, especially if you have specific health conditions or are taking medications. Daisy tea is known for its mild and soothing properties, making it a pleasant choice for relaxation and enjoyment.

Daisies, particularly the common daisy (Bellis perennis), are small flowering plants known for their bright and cheerful appearance. While they are not commonly used for medicinal or culinary purposes like some other herbs, daisies have various properties and uses:

1. Ornamental and Aesthetic:

- Daisies are primarily grown for their aesthetic value. They are popular ornamental flowers in gardens, flower arrangements, and floral decorations, often symbolizing innocence and purity.

2. Edible Flowers:

- While not widely consumed, daisy flowers are edible and can be used as a decorative element in salads, desserts, and beverages. They have a mild, slightly earthy taste.

3. Potential Healing Properties:

- In traditional herbal medicine, daisies have been used topically in various forms, such as poultices or ointments, for their potential soothing and anti-inflammatory properties. They may have been applied to minor skin irritations, bruises, and insect bites.

4. Potential Anti-Inflammatory Effects:

- Some anecdotal evidence suggests that daisies may have mild anti-inflammatory effects when applied topically. However, scientific research in this area is limited, and more studies are needed to confirm their effectiveness.

5. Folk Medicine:

- Daisies have a history of use in folk medicine for various purposes, including easing coughs, promoting wound healing, and relieving minor digestive discomfort. These uses are often based on traditional knowledge passed down through generations.

6. Pollinator-Friendly:

- Daisies are pollinator-friendly plants that attract bees, butterflies, and other beneficial insects to gardens. Their nectar-rich flowers provide food for these pollinators.

7. Lawn and Ground Cover:

- In some regions, particularly in Europe, daisies are considered desirable as part of a natural lawn or ground cover. They can create a charming and low-maintenance landscape.

8. Potential Herbal Tea Ingredient:

- While not as commonly used as other herbs, daisy flowers may be used in herbal tea blends for their mild floral flavour. These teas are often consumed for relaxation and their pleasant taste.

9. Cultural and Symbolic Significance:

- Daisies have cultural and symbolic significance in various societies. They are often associated with qualities like innocence, purity, and simplicity, and they appear in literature, art, and folklore.

10. Environmental Value: - Daisies contribute to biodiversity by providing habitat and food for insects. They are part of the natural ecosystem and play a role in maintaining environmental balance.

11. Easy-to-Grow Plant: - Daisies are generally easy to grow and are considered a beginner-friendly plant for gardeners. They thrive in a variety of soil types and climate conditions.

It's important to note that while daisies have various uses and properties, they are not typically relied upon as a primary source of medicine or nutrition. If you plan to use daisies for culinary or medicinal purposes, it's essential to positively identify the species and take any necessary precautions. Additionally, consult with a healthcare professional for any specific health-related concerns or treatments.

CHAMOMILE TEA

Chamomile tea is a soothing and calming herbal infusion known for its mild, floral flavour and potential health benefits. Here's a simple recipe to make a cup of chamomile tea:

Ingredients:

- 1 chamomile tea bag or 1 to 2 teaspoons of dried chamomile flowers (you can find chamomile tea bags and dried chamomile flowers at most grocery stores or online)
- 1 cup (8 ounces) of boiling water
- Honey or lemon (optional, for flavour)

Instructions:

- **Boil Water:**
  - Begin by bringing a cup of water (8 ounces) to a rolling boil. You can use a kettle or a saucepan for this purpose.
- **Prepare Chamomile Tea Bag or Dried Flowers:**
  - If you're using a chamomile tea bag, place it in your teacup. If you're using dried chamomile flowers, measure out 1 to 2 teaspoons of the dried flowers and place them in your teacup.
- **Pour Boiling Water:**
  - Carefully pour the freshly boiled water over the chamomile tea bag or dried flowers in your teacup.

- **Steep:**
    - Cover the teacup with a saucer or a small plate to trap the steam and essential oils and let the tea steep for about 5-7 minutes. This allows the flavours and beneficial compounds to infuse into the water.
- **Remove the Tea Bag or Strain (Optional):**
    - If you use a tea bag, simply remove it from the cup after the steeping time is up. If you used dried chamomile flowers, you can strain the tea as you pour it into another cup using a fine-mesh strainer to remove the flowers.
- **Optional Additions:**
    - If you like, you can sweeten your chamomile tea with honey to taste or add a squeeze of lemon for extra flavour. Chamomile tea has a mild, slightly floral taste, and these additions can enhance its palatability.
- **Serve:**
    - Your chamomile tea is now ready to enjoy. Sip it while it's still warm and take in the soothing and calming qualities of this herbal infusion.

Chamomile tea is often enjoyed before bedtime or as a gentle remedy for relaxation and stress relief. It's caffeine-free and has been associated with various potential health benefits, including aiding sleep, alleviating digestive discomfort, and reducing stress and anxiety. Chamomile tea is generally considered safe for most people, but if you have allergies to plants in the Asteraceae family (like ragweed), you may want to exercise caution or consult with a healthcare professional before consuming chamomile.

Chamomile, known for its botanical name Matricaria chamomilla (German chamomile) or Chamaemelum nobile (Roman chamomile), is an herb that offers a variety of properties and potential health benefits. Chamomile has been used for centuries in traditional medicine and herbal remedies due to its soothing and calming properties. Here are some of the notable properties and characteristics of chamomile:

1. Relaxing and Calming:

- Chamomile is perhaps best known for its calming and relaxation-inducing properties. It is often used to reduce stress, anxiety, and promote a sense of calm.

2. Aromatherapy:

- Chamomile essential oil is commonly used in aromatherapy to alleviate stress, improve sleep quality, and promote relaxation. It can be diffused, added to bathwater, or used in massage oils.

3. Sleep Aid:

- Chamomile is used as a natural remedy for sleep disorders. Drinking chamomile tea before bedtime is believed to improve sleep quality and alleviate insomnia.

4. Anti-Inflammatory:

- Chamomile possesses anti-inflammatory properties and may help reduce inflammation and related discomfort when applied topically or consumed as a tea.

5. Skin Health:

- Chamomile is known for its soothing effects on the skin. It is used in creams, ointments, and skincare products to alleviate skin irritations, minor burns, rashes, and insect bites.

6. Wound Healing:

- Chamomile promotes wound healing by stimulating tissue regeneration. It can be used topically to speed up the recovery of minor wounds and abrasions.

7. Antioxidant Content:

- Chamomile contains antioxidants, which help protect cells from oxidative stress and free radical damage. These antioxidants contribute to overall health.

8. Immune Support:

- Chamomile has immune-boosting properties and may help strengthen the body's defenses against infections and illnesses.

9. Digestive Aid:

- Chamomile tea is known to support digestion and alleviate symptoms of indigestion, gas, and bloating. It can also relieve gastrointestinal discomfort.

10. Respiratory Health: - Chamomile-infused steam inhalation or tea can help relieve respiratory discomfort, such as coughs, colds, and congestion.

11. Menstrual Health: - Chamomile tea is sometimes used to alleviate menstrual cramps and discomfort.

12. Gastrointestinal Health: - Chamomile tea may help soothe inflammation in the gastrointestinal tract and alleviate symptoms of conditions like gastritis.

13. Hair Care: - Chamomile-infused hair products can promote healthy hair and soothe scalp conditions like dandruff.

14. Culinary Uses: - Chamomile flowers are edible and can be used in culinary applications, including teas, desserts, and flavouring dishes.

15. Anti-Bacterial: - Chamomile has antibacterial properties, which can help prevent infections when applied topically or used as part of skincare routines.

16. Astringent: - Chamomile can be used as an astringent to help tighten and tone the skin.

Chamomile is available in various forms, including tea bags, dried flowers, essential oil, and skincare products. It is generally considered safe for most people when used as directed. However, if you have specific allergies or sensitivities, it's advisable to perform a patch test or consult with a healthcare professional before using chamomile products. Chamomile's soothing and calming properties make it a versatile herb, widely appreciated for its potential health benefits and natural healing properties.

CHAMOMILE, PASSIONFLOWER, MINT AND LEMON TEA

A chamomile, passionflower, mint and lemon tea is a delightful herbal blend that combines the soothing qualities of chamomile, the calming effects of passionflower, the refreshing taste of mint, and the citrusy zing of lemon. Here's a simple recipe to make this soothing and aromatic tea:

Ingredients:

- 1 chamomile tea bag or 1 to 2 teaspoons of dried chamomile flowers
- 1 passionflower tea bag or 1 to 2 teaspoons of dried passionflower leaves
- 1 peppermint tea bag or 1 to 2 teaspoons of dried peppermint leaves
- 1 slice of fresh lemon
- Honey (optional, for sweetness)
- 2 cups of boiling water

Instructions:

- **Boil Water:**
    - Start by boiling 2 cups (16 ounces) of water. You can use a kettle or a saucepan for this purpose.

- **Prepare the Herbs:**
    - If you're using tea bags for chamomile, passionflower, and peppermint, place them in your teapot or teacup. If you're using dried herbs, measure out 1 to 2 teaspoons of each herb and place them in your teapot or teacup.
- **Pour Boiling Water:**
    - Carefully pour the freshly boiled water over the tea bags or dried herbs in your teapot or teacup.
- **Add Lemon:**
    - Add a slice of fresh lemon to the teapot or teacup. The lemon will add a refreshing citrusy flavour to your tea.
- **Steep:**
    - Cover the teapot or teacup with a saucer or a small plate to trap the steam and essential oils and let the tea steep for about 5-7 minutes. This allows the flavours and properties of the herbs to infuse into the water. Adjust the steeping time to your taste, but avoid over-steeping, as it can make the tea too strong.
- **Remove Tea Bags (Optional):**
    - If you used tea bags, simply remove them from the teapot or teacup after the steeping time is up.
- **Optional Sweetener:**
    - If desired, add honey to taste for a touch of sweetness. This is entirely optional, as the lemon and mint can add natural flavour.
- **Serve:**
    - Your chamomile, passionflower, mint, and lemon tea is now ready to enjoy. Sip it while it's still warm and savour the soothing and calming qualities of this herbal blend.

This herbal tea combines the calming and relaxing properties of chamomile and passionflower with the refreshing and digestive benefits of peppermint and the zesty brightness of lemon. It's a wonderful choice for winding down before bedtime, reducing stress and anxiety, or simply enjoying a moment of tranquillity.

Passionflower (Passiflora incarnata) is a climbing vine with striking, intricate flowers that is known for its potential therapeutic properties.

The plant has a long history of use in traditional herbal medicine, particularly among Indigenous cultures in the Americas. Here are some of the notable properties and characteristics of passionflower:

1. Calming and Relaxing:

- Passionflower is perhaps best known for its calming and sedative properties. It has a soothing effect on the nervous system and can help reduce stress, anxiety, and restlessness. It is often used as a natural remedy for insomnia and improving sleep quality.

2. Aids Sleep:

- Passionflower is used to treat sleep disorders, including insomnia. It can help individuals fall asleep faster, sleep more soundly, and wake up feeling refreshed.

3. Anxiolytic (Anti-Anxiety):

- Passionflower has anxiolytic effects, which means it may reduce symptoms of anxiety and promote relaxation without causing drowsiness.

4. Mild Sedative:

- Passionflower acts as a mild sedative, which can be particularly helpful for individuals who experience nervousness or restlessness.

5. Muscle Relaxant:

- It has muscle relaxant properties and may help ease muscle tension and discomfort, including headaches caused by muscle tension.

6. Antioxidant Content:

- Passionflower contains antioxidants, which help protect cells from oxidative stress and free radical damage. Antioxidants are beneficial for overall health.

7. Gastrointestinal Support:

- Passionflower is sometimes used to alleviate digestive discomfort, including symptoms of indigestion and irritable bowel syndrome (IBS).

8. Menstrual and Menopausal Support:

- It may help reduce symptoms associated with menstruation and menopause, such as cramps, irritability, and hot flashes.

9. Anti-Inflammatory:

- Some studies suggest that passionflower may have anti-inflammatory properties, potentially benefiting conditions characterized by inflammation.

10. Potential Pain Relief: - Passionflower may offer mild pain-relieving properties and can help alleviate minor aches and pains.

11. Cardiovascular Health: - Some research suggests that passionflower may have a positive impact on heart health by helping to lower blood pressure and improve circulation.

12. Antispasmodic: - It has antispasmodic effects, which can help reduce muscle spasms and cramps.

13. Supports Cognitive Function: - Passionflower may have a positive effect on cognitive function, including memory and concentration.

14. Antiviral: - Some studies have explored passionflower's potential antiviral properties, though more research is needed to confirm its efficacy in this regard.

Passionflower is available in various forms, including herbal teas, tinctures, capsules, and as a dried herb for infusion. It is generally considered safe for most people when used as directed. However, it's advisable to consult with a healthcare professional before using passionflower, especially if you are pregnant, nursing, or taking medications, as there may be potential interactions or contraindications in some cases. Passionflower's calming and soothing properties have made it a popular herbal remedy for reducing anxiety and promoting relaxation.

MINT TEA

Mint tea is a delightful herbal infusion known for its refreshing and soothing properties. It can be made with various types of mint, such as peppermint or spearmint. Here's a simple recipe for making mint tea:

Ingredients:

- Fresh mint leaves (about 10-12 leaves per cup of tea) or 1-2 teaspoons of dried mint leaves per cup
- 1 cup of boiling water per serving
- Optional additions: honey, lemon, or other herbs for flavour

Instructions:

- **Prepare the Mint Leaves:**
    - If you're using fresh mint, gently wash the mint leaves under cold running water to remove any dirt or debris. For dried mint, measure out 1-2 teaspoons per cup of tea.
- **Boil Water:**
    - Boil the desired amount of water in a kettle or on the stovetop. You'll need about one cup (8 ounces) of boiling water per serving of mint tea.

- **Place Mint Leaves in a Cup:**
  - If using fresh mint, place 10-12 leaves into a teacup or teapot. If using dried mint, add 1-2 teaspoons of dried mint leaves per cup.
- **Pour Boiling Water:**
  - Carefully pour the boiling water over the mint leaves. Make sure the leaves are fully submerged.
- **Steep:**
  - Allow the mint leaves to steep in the hot water for about 5-7 minutes. You can adjust the steeping time to your taste, but be cautious not to over-steep, as mint tea can become quite strong if left too long.
- **Optional Additions:**
  - If desired, you can sweeten your mint tea with honey or add a squeeze of lemon for extra flavour. Mint tea has a naturally refreshing taste, and these additions can complement it.
- **Strain (Optional):**
  - If you prefer not to have mint leaves in your tea, use a fine-mesh strainer to remove the leaves while pouring the tea into your cup.
- **Enjoy:**
  - Your mint tea is now ready to enjoy. Sip it while it's still warm.

Mint tea is a simple and versatile beverage. You can adjust the strength of the mint flavour by using more or fewer leaves and varying the steeping time. It's a wonderful choice for relaxation and digestion, and it can be served both hot and cold, making it suitable for different seasons and occasions.

Fresh mint, whether it's peppermint or spearmint, is a versatile herb that offers various properties and potential health benefits. Here are some of the key properties and characteristics of fresh mint:

1. Refreshing Flavour:

- Fresh mint has a refreshing and invigorating flavour with a cool, slightly sweet, and mildly pungent taste. Its aromatic qualities make it a popular addition to both culinary and beverage recipes.

2. Aromatic Compounds:

- Mint leaves contain aromatic compounds, including menthol (more prominent in peppermint) and carvone (more prominent in spearmint), which contribute to their distinctive scent and flavour.

3. Digestive Aid:

- Mint has a long history of use as a digestive aid. It may help relieve indigestion, bloating, and gas. Drinking mint tea or chewing mint leaves after a meal is a common practice for promoting digestion.

4. Natural Breath Freshener:

- The antibacterial properties of mint can help freshen breath. Chewing on fresh mint leaves or using mint-based chewing gum or breath mints can temporarily mask bad breath.

5. Potential Anti-Nausea Effects:

- Mint, particularly peppermint, is sometimes used to alleviate nausea and motion sickness. It may help relax the muscles in the gastrointestinal tract and reduce feelings of queasiness.

6. Headache Relief:

- The menthol in mint can have a soothing effect on headaches. Applying diluted peppermint oil to the temples or inhaling its vapor may provide relief for some individuals.

7. Stress Reduction:

- The aroma of mint is known for its potential stress-reducing and calming effects. It can help create a sense of relaxation and mental clarity.

8. Potential Anti-Inflammatory Properties:

- Mint contains compounds with potential anti-inflammatory properties, which may help reduce inflammation and discomfort associated with conditions like arthritis.

9. Antioxidant Content:

- Mint leaves are a source of antioxidants, which can help protect cells from oxidative stress and damage caused by free radicals.

10. Skin Care: - Mint extracts and essential oils are used in skincare products for their potential benefits. They may help soothe irritated skin, reduce itchiness, and provide a cooling sensation.

11. Culinary Versatility: - Fresh mint is a versatile herb used in various culinary dishes and beverages. It pairs well with both sweet and savoury flavours and is commonly used in salads, sauces, desserts, and beverages like mint tea, mojitos, and mint juleps.

12. Home Remedies: - Mint is used in home remedies and natural remedies for various ailments, from treating insect bites to soothing sunburned skin.

13. Herbal Infusions: - Mint leaves can be used to make herbal infusions or teas, which are known for their soothing properties and pleasant flavour.

14. Easy to Grow: - Mint is a hardy herb that is easy to grow in home gardens or pots. It tends to thrive in a variety of climates and conditions.

It's important to note that while fresh mint offers numerous potential benefits, individual responses can vary. If you have specific health concerns or medical conditions, consult with a healthcare professional before using mint for medicinal purposes. Additionally, some individuals may be sensitive to mint or menthol, so it's essential to use mint products in moderation.

PEPPERMINT, GINGER, LEMON AND BLACK TEA

Peppermint, ginger, lemon, and black tea can be combined to create a flavourful and aromatic tea blend that offers a refreshing and soothing experience. Here's a simple recipe for peppermint ginger lemon black tea:

Ingredients:

- 1 black tea bag or 1 to 2 teaspoons of loose black tea leaves
- 1 peppermint tea bag or 1 to 2 teaspoons of dried peppermint leaves
- 1 slice of fresh ginger (about 1/4 inch thick)
- 1 slice of fresh lemon
- Honey (optional, for sweetness)
- 2 cups of boiling water

Instructions:

- **Boil Water:**
    - Start by boiling 2 cups (16 ounces) of water. You can use a kettle or a saucepan for this purpose.
- **Prepare the Tea:**
    - Place the black tea bag or loose black tea leaves in your teapot or teacup. If you're using loose tea leaves, you may want to use a tea strainer.
- **Add Peppermint:**
    - Add the peppermint tea bag or dried peppermint leaves to the teapot or teacup with the black tea.

- **Add Ginger:**
    - Add the fresh ginger slice to the teapot or teacup. Ginger adds a warming and slightly spicy flavour to the tea.
- **Add Lemon:**
    - Add a slice of fresh lemon to the teapot or teacup. The lemon will infuse the tea with a bright and citrusy aroma.
- **Pour Boiling Water:**
    - Carefully pour the freshly boiled water over the tea bags or tea leaves, ginger, and lemon in your teapot or teacup.
- **Steep:**
    - Cover the teapot or teacup with a saucer or a small plate to trap the steam and essential oils and let the tea steep for about 3-5 minutes. This allows the flavours and properties of the herbs to infuse into the water. Adjust the steeping time to your taste.
- **Remove Tea Bags (Optional):**
    - If you used tea bags, simply remove them from the teapot or teacup after the steeping time is up.
- **Optional Sweetener:**
    - If desired, add honey to taste for a touch of sweetness. This is entirely optional, as the lemon and mint can add natural flavour.
- **Serve:**
    - Your peppermint ginger lemon black tea is now ready to enjoy. Sip it while it's still warm and savour the delightful blend of flavours and the potential health benefits of this herbal-infused black tea.

This tea combines the robust and slightly astringent taste of black tea with the refreshing qualities of peppermint, the spicy warmth of ginger, and the zesty brightness of lemon. It's an invigorating choice for any time of day and can be enjoyed both hot and cold. Plus, each of these ingredients brings its own potential health benefits, making this tea blend a soothing and flavourful option.

ECHINACEA TEA

Echinacea tea is an herbal infusion made from the dried leaves, flowers, and roots of the echinacea plant, primarily Echinacea purpurea and Echinacea angustifolia. Echinacea, also known as purple coneflower, is a popular herb in traditional and alternative medicine due to its potential health benefits. Here's an overview of echinacea tea:

Preparation:

- To make echinacea tea, you can use either echinacea tea bags or dried echinacea plant parts (leaves, flowers, and roots). Here's how to prepare it:
    - Boil water and let it cool slightly (about 200°F or 93°C).
    - Place 1 to 2 teaspoons of dried echinacea or one echinacea tea bag in a teapot or cup.
    - Pour the hot water over the echinacea.
    - Cover and steep for about 10-15 minutes to allow the echinacea to infuse into the water.

Flavour:

- Echinacea tea has a slightly earthy, floral, and mildly bitter flavour. Some people find it pleasant, while others may add honey or lemon to enhance the taste.

Caution and Considerations:

- While echinacea is generally considered safe for short-term use, it's essential to exercise caution and consult with a healthcare professional, especially if you have allergies, are pregnant, nursing, or taking medications.
- It's recommended to limit the use of echinacea to a few weeks at a time and take breaks to avoid potential side effects or reduced effectiveness.

Echinacea tea can be a soothing and potentially beneficial beverage, especially during cold and flu seasons or when you need immune support.

However, it's important to use it as part of a well-rounded approach to health and consult with a healthcare provider for personalized advice, particularly if you have underlying health conditions or concerns.

Echinacea, also known as purple coneflower, is a popular herbal remedy known for its potential health benefits. It has been used for centuries in traditional medicine, primarily by Indigenous people in North America. Echinacea is available in various forms, including supplements, tinctures, and teas, and is believed to possess several properties and potential therapeutic effects. Here are some of the notable properties and characteristics of echinacea:

1. Immune-Boosting: Echinacea is best known for its immune-enhancing properties. It is believed to stimulate the production and activity of immune cells, helping the body defend against infections, particularly colds and respiratory illnesses. Many people use echinacea as a natural remedy to reduce the severity and duration of cold symptoms.

2. Anti-Inflammatory: Echinacea has anti-inflammatory properties, which can help reduce inflammation in the body. This can be beneficial for conditions characterized by inflammation, such as arthritis and skin irritations.

3. Antioxidant Content: Echinacea contains antioxidants, including flavonoids and polyphenols, which help protect cells from oxidative stress and free radical damage. Antioxidants contribute to overall health and may play a role in disease prevention.

4. Antiviral and Antibacterial: Some research suggests that echinacea may have antiviral and antibacterial properties, making it potentially useful for preventing and managing infections caused by viruses and bacteria.

5. Respiratory Health: Echinacea is often used to alleviate symptoms of respiratory infections, such as coughs, bronchitis, and sinusitis. It may help reduce congestion and inflammation in the respiratory tract.

6. Wound Healing: Echinacea is used topically to promote wound healing and alleviate skin irritations, minor burns, and insect bites. It can be applied as a cream, ointment, or gel.

7. Potential Cancer Support: Some studies have explored the potential of echinacea in cancer prevention and treatment due to its immune-boosting and anti-inflammatory properties. However, more research is needed in this area.

8. Allergy Relief: Echinacea may help alleviate symptoms of allergies, such as hay fever, by reducing inflammation and modulating the immune response.

9. Adaptogenic: Echinacea is considered an adaptogen, which means it may help the body adapt to stress and maintain balance.

10. Mild Analgesic: Echinacea may have mild pain-relieving properties and can help reduce minor aches and pains.

11. Blood Sugar Regulation: Some research has suggested that echinacea may help regulate blood sugar levels, which can be beneficial for individuals with diabetes.

12. Cardiovascular Health: Echinacea may have a positive impact on heart health by helping to lower blood pressure and reduce the risk of heart disease.

It's important to note that while echinacea is generally considered safe for short-term use, there can be variations in the quality and effectiveness of echinacea products. Additionally, some people may experience side effects or allergic reactions, so it's advisable to consult with a healthcare professional before using echinacea, especially if you have specific health concerns, allergies, or are taking medications. Echinacea's immune-boosting and anti-inflammatory properties have made it a popular choice for immune support and overall well-being.

ECHINACEA, ELDERBERRY AND LEMON TEA

Echinacea, elderberry, and lemon tea is a delightful herbal blend that combines the immune-boosting properties of echinacea and elderberry with the zesty brightness of lemon. This tea can be soothing, comforting, and potentially beneficial for supporting your immune system, particularly during cold and flu seasons. Here's a simple recipe to make this herbal tea:

Ingredients:

- 1 echinacea tea bag or 1 to 2 teaspoons of dried echinacea leaves and flowers
- 1 elderberry tea bag or 1 to 2 teaspoons of dried elderberry
- 1 slice of fresh lemon
- Honey (optional, for sweetness)
- 2 cups of boiling water

Instructions:

- **Boil Water:**
    - Start by boiling 2 cups (16 ounces) of water. You can use a kettle or a saucepan for this purpose.
- **Prepare the Tea:**
    - Place the echinacea tea bag or dried echinacea leaves and flowers in your teapot or teacup. If you're using loose tea leaves, you may want to use a tea strainer.
- **Add Elderberry:**
    - Add the elderberry tea bag or dried elderberries to the teapot or teacup with the echinacea.
- **Add Lemon:**
    - Add a slice of fresh lemon to the teapot or teacup. The lemon will infuse the tea with a bright and citrusy aroma.
- **Pour Boiling Water:**
    - Carefully pour the freshly boiled water over the tea bags or tea leaves, elderberry, and lemon in your teapot or teacup.
- **Steep:**
    - Cover the teapot or teacup with a saucer or a small plate to trap the steam and essential oils and let the tea steep for about 5-7 minutes. This allows the flavours and properties of the herbs to infuse into the water. Adjust the steeping time to your taste.

- **Remove Tea Bags (Optional):**
    - If you used tea bags, simply remove them from the teapot or teacup after the steeping time is up.
- **Optional Sweetener:**
    - If desired, add honey to taste for a touch of sweetness. This is entirely optional, as the lemon and elderberry can add natural flavour.
- **Serve:**
    - Your echinacea, elderberry, and lemon tea is now ready to enjoy. Sip it while it's still warm and savour the delightful blend of flavours and the potential immune-boosting benefits of this herbal-infused tea.

This herbal tea combines the immune-enhancing properties of echinacea and elderberry with the refreshing citrus notes of lemon. It's a comforting choice for promoting overall well-being and providing support during times of immune system challenges. Plus, it's a delicious way to enjoy the potential health benefits of these herbal ingredients.

If you're not a big fan of black tea, you can use green tea to combine with all the other tea ingredients. It will taste different but it will be delicious. Green tea is a popular beverage made from the leaves of the Camellia sinensis plant. It is well-known for its potential health benefits and is rich in various bioactive compounds. Here are some of the notable properties and characteristics of green tea:

1. Antioxidant-Rich: Green tea is loaded with antioxidants, particularly catechins, which help protect cells from oxidative stress and free radical damage. Epigallocatechin gallate (EGCG) is the most abundant and potent catechin in green tea.

2. Cardiovascular Health: Green tea consumption has been associated with a reduced risk of cardiovascular diseases. It may help lower levels of bad LDL cholesterol and improve overall cholesterol profiles.

3. Weight Management: Green tea is believed to boost metabolism and fat oxidation, making it a popular choice for those looking to manage their weight. It may also help reduce abdominal fat.

4. Brain Health: The caffeine and L-theanine in green tea can enhance brain function and improve alertness, memory, and cognitive performance. They work synergistically to provide a calm but alert mental state.

5. Cancer Prevention: Some studies suggest that the antioxidants in green tea, particularly EGCG, may help protect against certain types of cancer by inhibiting the growth of cancer cells.

6. Anti-Inflammatory: Green tea has anti-inflammatory properties that can help reduce inflammation in the body. Chronic inflammation is linked to various diseases, including arthritis.

7. Immune Support: The catechins in green tea may enhance the immune system's function, helping the body fight off infections and illnesses.

8. Oral Health: Green tea contains fluoride and antibacterial compounds that can help reduce the growth of harmful bacteria in the mouth, improving oral health and reducing the risk of cavities and bad breath.

9. Skin Benefits: The antioxidants in green tea can help protect the skin from UV radiation damage, reduce signs of aging, and promote a healthy complexion. Green tea extracts are used in various skincare products.

10. Diabetes Management: Some studies have suggested that green tea may help regulate blood sugar levels and improve insulin sensitivity, making it potentially beneficial for individuals with diabetes.

11. Relaxation and Stress Reduction: L-theanine, an amino acid found in green tea, promotes relaxation and reduces stress without causing drowsiness. It can help reduce anxiety and improve overall mood.

12. Liver Health: Green tea may support liver function and help protect the liver from damage caused by alcohol consumption and certain toxins.

13. Anti-Bacterial: Green tea has natural antibacterial properties that can help prevent infections and promote oral and digestive health.

14. Anti-Viral: Some research suggests that green tea catechins may have antiviral properties, which can be helpful in fighting common viral infections.

It's important to note that the specific health benefits of green tea can vary depending on the type of green tea, the quality, and the preparation method. Drinking green tea as part of a balanced diet and healthy lifestyle may contribute to overall well-being. However, it's advisable to moderate your consumption, as excessive intake of caffeine from green tea can have side effects, such as insomnia and digestive upset. Additionally, if you have specific health concerns or are taking medications, it's a good idea to consult with a healthcare professional before making green tea a regular part of your diet.

ROSEHIP, HIBISCUS AND CHERRY TEA

Rosehip, hibiscus, and cherry tea is a delightful and vibrant herbal blend that combines the fruity flavours of rosehips and cherries with the tartness of hibiscus. This tea is not only flavourful but also packed with antioxidants and potential health benefits. Here's a simple recipe to make this colorful and tasty herbal tea:

Ingredients:

- 2 tablespoons of dried rosehips
- 2 tablespoons of dried hibiscus flowers
- 1 tablespoon of dried cherries (or cherry pieces)
- Honey or agave nectar (optional, for sweetness)
- 4 cups of boiling water

Instructions:

- **Boil Water:**
  - Start by bringing 4 cups (32 ounces) of water to a boil in a kettle or saucepan.
- **Prepare the Tea Blend:**
  - In a teapot or heatproof container, combine the dried rosehips, dried hibiscus flowers, and dried cherries.

These are the key ingredients that will infuse the tea with their flavours and health benefits.

- **Pour Boiling Water:**
    - Carefully pour the boiling water over the tea blend in your teapot or container.
- **Steep:**
    - Cover the teapot or container with a lid or a saucer to trap the steam and aroma. Let the tea steep for about 5-7 minutes. Adjust the steeping time to your taste, but be cautious not to over-steep, as hibiscus can become quite tart if steeped for too long.
- **Strain:**
    - If you used loose tea leaves, strain the tea into cups or a serving teapot to remove the solid ingredients.
- **Optional Sweetener:**
    - If desired, add honey or agave nectar to sweeten the tea to your liking. Taste and adjust as needed.
- **Serve:**
    - Your rosehip, hibiscus, and cherry tea is now ready to enjoy. Serve it hot and savour the vibrant flavours and potential health benefits of this herbal blend.

This tea offers a delightful combination of tartness from the hibiscus, fruity notes from the rosehips and cherries, and the option to sweeten it to your preference. It's rich in vitamin C and antioxidants, making it a refreshing and healthful choice. Plus, it can be enjoyed both hot and cold, making it suitable for various occasions and seasons.

EUCALYPTUS TEA

Eucalyptus tea is a herbal infusion made from the leaves of the eucalyptus tree. It is known for its refreshing and soothing qualities, as well as potential health benefits, especially for respiratory health. Here's a simple recipe to make eucalyptus tea:

Ingredients:

- 1 to 2 teaspoons of dried eucalyptus leaves (or 1 eucalyptus tea bag)
- 1 cup of boiling water
- Honey or lemon (optional, for flavour)

Instructions:

- **Boil Water:**
    - Start by boiling 1 cup (8 ounces) of water. You can use a kettle or a saucepan for this purpose.
- **Prepare the Tea:**
    - Place the dried eucalyptus leaves or eucalyptus tea bag in a teapot or teacup.
- **Pour Boiling Water:**
    - Carefully pour the freshly boiled water over the eucalyptus leaves or tea bag in your teapot or teacup.
- **Steep:**
    - Cover the teapot or teacup with a saucer or a small plate to trap the steam and essential oils and let the tea steep for about 5-7 minutes. This allows the flavours and properties of the eucalyptus leaves to infuse into the water. Adjust the steeping time to your taste.
- **Remove Tea Bag (If used):**
    - If you use a tea bag, simply remove it from the teapot or teacup after the steeping time is up.
- **Optional Flavour Additions:**
    - If desired, you can add honey or a squeeze of lemon to your eucalyptus tea for additional flavour. These additions can also provide extra soothing qualities to the tea.
- **Serve:**
    - Your eucalyptus tea is now ready to enjoy. Sip it while it's still warm and savour the refreshing and invigorating qualities of this herbal infusion.

Eucalyptus tea has a fresh, clean, and slightly minty flavour. It's particularly appreciated for its potential respiratory benefits, as it can help alleviate congestion and soothe sore throats. Additionally, eucalyptus tea is often used to relieve symptoms of colds and flu.

Please note that while eucalyptus tea is generally safe, it's crucial to use it in moderation and consult with a healthcare professional if you have specific health concerns or are pregnant, nursing, or taking medications. As with any herbal remedy, individual responses may vary, and it's essential to use eucalyptus tea responsibly for its intended purposes.

Eucalyptus is a diverse genus of trees and shrubs, primarily native to Australia but also found in other parts of the world. Eucalyptus species are known for their aromatic leaves and have been used for various purposes, including traditional medicine and industrial applications. Here are some of the notable properties and characteristics of eucalyptus:

1. Aromatic: Eucalyptus leaves contain essential oils with a strong, distinctive aroma. This aroma is often described as fresh, camphoraceous, and minty. The scent of eucalyptus is invigorating and is used in various products, including essential oils, perfumes, and cleaning products.

2. Medicinal: Eucalyptus has been used for centuries in traditional medicine, primarily for its potential health benefits, including:

- **Respiratory Health:** Eucalyptus is known for its ability to relieve respiratory symptoms. Inhalation of eucalyptus essential oil or steam from eucalyptus-infused water can help alleviate congestion, coughs, and sinusitis.
- **Anti-Inflammatory:** Eucalyptus may have anti-inflammatory properties and can be used topically to reduce inflammation and soothe skin irritations.
- **Antiseptic and Antibacterial:** Eucalyptus oil is an effective antiseptic and has antibacterial properties. It's often used in topical applications to clean wounds and prevent infection.
- **Analgesic:** Eucalyptus oil can act as a mild pain reliever when applied topically to sore muscles and joints.

3. Respiratory Benefits: Eucalyptus is commonly used in cough drops, throat lozenges, and chest rubs to help relieve respiratory discomfort and promote easier breathing.

4. Essential Oil: Eucalyptus essential oil is extracted from the leaves and is used in aromatherapy for its soothing and decongestant properties. It's often diffused in the air or added to steam inhalations.

5. Industrial Uses: Eucalyptus wood is valued for its durability and is used in construction, furniture, and paper production. Eucalyptus oil is also used in the perfume, cosmetics, and fragrance industries.

6. Insect Repellent: Eucalyptus oil can act as a natural insect repellent and is used in mosquito repellent products.

7. Environmental Impact: Eucalyptus trees are known for their rapid growth and adaptability to various climates. They are sometimes planted for reforestation and timber production.

8. Culinary Uses: Some species of eucalyptus produce edible seeds, flowers, and leaves. In Australia, Indigenous people have used certain parts of eucalyptus trees for food.

9. Eucalyptus Varieties: There are hundreds of eucalyptus species, each with their unique properties and uses. The oil extracted from different species can vary in chemical composition and aroma.

It's important to note that while eucalyptus offers numerous benefits, the use of eucalyptus essential oil should be done with care. Essential oils are highly concentrated and should be diluted properly before topical application. Additionally, eucalyptus oil should not be ingested unless under the guidance of a qualified healthcare professional. Always consult with a healthcare provider or aromatherapist before using eucalyptus products, especially if you have specific health concerns or are pregnant, nursing, or taking medications.

ROSE TEA

Rose tea is a delightful herbal infusion made from the petals of roses. It has a delicate, floral aroma and a subtly sweet taste. Rose tea can be made from fresh rose petals or dried rose petals and is enjoyed for both its pleasant flavour and potential health benefits. Here's a simple recipe for making rose tea using dried rose petals:

Ingredients:

- 1 to 2 teaspoons of dried rose petals
- 1 cup of boiling water
- Optional additions: honey or a slice of lemon for flavour

Instructions:

- **Prepare the Dried Rose Petals:**
  - Measure out 1 to 2 teaspoons of dried rose petals per cup of tea. You can adjust the amount based on your preference for a stronger or milder flavour.
- **Boil Water:**
  - Bring one cup (8 ounces) of water to a boil in a kettle or on the stovetop.
- **Place Dried Rose Petals in a Cup:**
  - Put the dried rose petals into a teacup or teapot.
- **Pour Boiling Water:**
  - Carefully pour the boiling water over the dried rose petals, ensuring they are fully submerged.
- **Steep:**
  - Allow the dried rose petals to steep in the hot water for about 5-7 minutes. You can adjust the steeping time to your taste, but avoid over-steeping, as it can make the tea overly floral.
- **Optional Additions:**
  - If desired, you can sweeten your rose tea with honey or add a slice of lemon for extra flavour. Rose tea has a naturally gentle and floral taste, and these additions can enhance its overall profile.

- **Strain (Optional):**
  - If you prefer not to have rose petals in your tea, use a fine-mesh strainer to remove them while pouring the tea into your cup.
- **Enjoy:**
  - Your rose tea is now ready to enjoy. Sip it while it's still warm.

Note: Rose tea is generally considered safe for most people and is caffeine-free. It's known for its potential to promote relaxation and reduce stress due to its pleasant aroma and calming properties. Additionally, rose tea may contain antioxidants, which can have various health benefits. However, if you have specific allergies or sensitivities, it's a good idea to check with a healthcare professional before consuming rose tea regularly. Additionally, when making rose tea, ensure that you are using roses specifically grown for culinary or tea purposes, as some roses may be treated with pesticides or other chemicals not suitable for consumption.

Rose tea, made from the petals of roses, is celebrated for its delicate flavour and potential health benefits. Here are some of the properties and characteristics of rose tea:

1. Delicate Floral Flavour:

- Rose tea has a mild, sweet, and floral flavour. The aroma and taste are reminiscent of fresh roses, providing a soothing and pleasant experience.

2. Aromatic Qualities:

- The aroma of rose tea is calming and can be used for relaxation and stress relief. Inhaling the scent of rose petals can have a soothing effect on the mind and emotions.

3. Caffeine-Free:

- Rose tea is naturally caffeine-free, making it an excellent choice for those looking to avoid or reduce caffeine intake.

4. Potential Antioxidants:

- Roses, particularly petals, contain antioxidants that help protect cells from oxidative stress and free radical damage. Antioxidants may have various health benefits.

5. Hydration:

- Rose tea, like other herbal infusions, can contribute to daily hydration, which is essential for overall health and well-being.

6. Potential Anti-Inflammatory Properties:

- Some studies suggest that rose petals may have anti-inflammatory properties, which can be beneficial for reducing inflammation and related discomfort.

7. Skin Health:

- The antioxidants in rose tea may promote healthy skin by protecting against premature aging and helping to maintain skin's natural glow. Rosewater, a byproduct of rose petal distillation, is often used in skincare products.

8. Digestive Aid:

- Rose tea is traditionally used to support digestion and soothe digestive discomfort. It may help alleviate symptoms of indigestion, bloating, and upset stomach.

9. Menstrual Health:

- Rose tea is sometimes consumed by women for its potential benefits in easing menstrual discomfort and promoting hormonal balance.

10. Calming Effect: - The aroma and taste of rose tea are known for their calming and stress-relieving properties. It can be enjoyed as part of a relaxation routine or to unwind after a long day.

11. Potential Respiratory Benefits: - Rose tea may provide relief from respiratory discomfort and soothe sore throats when consumed warm.

12. Culinary Uses: - Dried rose petals can be used as a culinary ingredient in various recipes, including desserts, jams, and confections. They can add a subtle floral note to dishes.

13. Emotional Well-Being: - In some cultures, rose tea is associated with emotional well-being and can be used in rituals and ceremonies to promote positive feelings and connection.

14. Soothing Sore Throats: - Gargling with rose tea may provide relief for sore throats due to its mild astringent properties.

It's important to note that while rose tea offers potential health benefits, individual responses can vary. Additionally, it's advisable to use roses that are specifically grown for culinary or tea purposes, as some roses may be treated with pesticides or other chemicals not suitable for consumption. If you have specific allergies or are pregnant, it's a good idea to consult with a healthcare professional before consuming rose tea regularly.

RED CLOVER TEA

Red clover tea is an herbal infusion made from the dried flowers or leaves of the red clover plant (Trifolium pratense). Red clover is a legume native to Europe and Asia but is now grown in various parts of the world. The plant is known for its potential health benefits, and its tea is often consumed for its mild, sweet flavour and potential therapeutic properties. Here's how to make red clover tea:

Ingredients:

- 1 to 2 tablespoons of dried red clover flowers or leaves
- 1 cup of boiling water
- Honey or lemon (optional, for flavour)

Instructions:

- **Boil Water:**
    - Start by bringing 1 cup (8 ounces) of water to a boil in a kettle or saucepan.
- **Prepare the Tea:**
    - Place the dried red clover flowers or leaves in a teapot or teacup. You can use a tea strainer or an infuser to contain the loose tea if you prefer.
- **Pour Boiling Water:**
    - Carefully pour the boiling water over the red clover flowers or leaves in your teapot or teacup.
- **Steep:**
    - Cover the teapot or teacup with a lid or a saucer to trap the steam and aroma. Let the tea steep for about 5-10 minutes. Adjust the steeping time to your taste; longer steeping may result in a stronger flavour.
- **Strain (If needed):**
    - If you used loose red clover flowers or leaves, strain the tea into a cup to remove the solid ingredients.
- **Optional Flavour Additions:**
    - If desired, you can add honey or a squeeze of lemon to your red clover tea for additional flavour. These additions can enhance the taste and add natural sweetness.
- **Serve:**
    - Your red clover tea is now ready to enjoy. Sip it while it's still warm and savour the mild, slightly sweet flavour of this herbal infusion.

Red clover tea is known for its potential health benefits, which include:

1. Phytoestrogens: Red clover contains compounds called isoflavones, which are known as phytoestrogens. These compounds may have a mild estrogen-like effect in the body and have been studied for their potential benefits in managing menopausal symptoms.

2. Antioxidants: Red clover is rich in antioxidants, which help protect cells from oxidative stress and free radical damage. Antioxidants contribute to overall health and may play a role in disease prevention.

3. Skin Health: Some people use red clover tea topically to soothe skin irritations and promote healthy skin.

4. Respiratory Health: Red clover tea is believed to have mild respiratory benefits and may help soothe coughs and cold symptoms.

5. Nutrient-Rich: Red clover contains essential nutrients such as vitamins and minerals, including calcium, magnesium, and vitamin C.

As with any herbal remedy, it's essential to use red clover tea in moderation, and it's advisable to consult with a healthcare professional if you have specific health concerns or are pregnant, nursing, or taking medications. While red clover tea is generally considered safe for most people when consumed as a beverage, individual responses may vary. Enjoying red clover tea as part of a balanced diet and healthy lifestyle can be a pleasant way to explore its potential benefits.

As you can see you can put ALMOST anything in your teapot, but please, always check if it's safe before doing so.

I've always liked fruit teas, so I decided to impress myself and my guests at one of my friends' visits and I made strawberry iced tea. It was a hit!

STRAWBERRY ICED TEA

Dried strawberry iced tea is a refreshing and fruity beverage perfect for warm weather. It combines the sweet and tangy flavours of dried strawberries with the refreshing qualities of iced tea. Here's a simple recipe to make your own dried strawberry iced tea:

Ingredients:

- 4 cups of water
- 4 black tea bags (or your favorite tea variety)
- 1/2 cup of dried strawberries
- 1/4 cup of sugar (adjust to taste)
- Ice cubes
- Fresh strawberry slices (optional, for garnish)
- Lemon slices (optional, for garnish)
- Fresh mint leaves (optional, for garnish)

Instructions:

- **Prepare the Tea:**
    - Bring 4 cups of water to a boil in a pot. Once boiling, remove it from heat and add the tea bags. Allow the tea to steep for about 5-7 minutes, or according to the package instructions, to achieve your desired tea strength.
- **Sweeten the Tea:**
    - While the tea is still hot, stir in the sugar until it dissolves completely. You can adjust the amount of sugar to your taste. If you prefer a sweeter tea, you can add more sugar.
- **Add the Dried Strawberries:**
    - Place the dried strawberries in a separate heatproof container or teapot. Pour the hot tea over the dried strawberries. This will rehydrate the strawberries and

infuse the tea with their fruity flavour. Allow this mixture
to steep for an additional 10-15 minutes.

- **Strain and Cool:**
  - After steeping, strain the tea to remove the tea bags and
    any solid pieces, such as rehydrated strawberry bits.
    Allow the tea to cool to room temperature, and then
    refrigerate it until it's thoroughly chilled.
- **Serve:**
  - Fill glasses with ice cubes and pour the chilled
    strawberry-infused tea over the ice.
- **Garnish (Optional):**
  - Garnish your iced tea with fresh strawberry slices, lemon
    slices, and mint leaves for an extra burst of flavour and a
    visually appealing presentation.
- **Enjoy:**
  - Serve your dried strawberry iced tea immediately and
    enjoy it on a hot day as a refreshing and fruity beverage.

Feel free to adjust the sweetness and the strength of the strawberry
flavour by varying the amount of sugar and dried strawberries you use.
You can also experiment with different tea varieties to find your favorite
combination. Green tea or herbal tea blends can be excellent choices for
a unique twist on this refreshing drink.

Dried strawberries are a convenient and delicious snack made by
removing the moisture from fresh strawberries. They retain much of the
flavour and many of the nutrients found in fresh strawberries, along with
some unique characteristics. Here are some of the properties and
characteristics of dried strawberries:

1. Sweet and Intense Flavour:

- Dried strawberries have a concentrated, sweet, and fruity
  flavour. The drying process amplifies the natural sugars in the
  strawberries, making them taste even sweeter compared to their
  fresh counterparts.

2. Nutrient Retention:

- Drying strawberries preserves many of the vitamins and minerals found in fresh strawberries. They are particularly rich in vitamin C, which is known for its antioxidant properties and immune system support.

3. Antioxidant Content:

- Dried strawberries contain antioxidants, including anthocyanins and quercetin, which help combat oxidative stress and protect cells from free radical damage.

4. Dietary Fiber:

- Dried strawberries are a source of dietary fiber, which can aid in digestion and help maintain regular bowel movements.

5. Convenience:

- Dried strawberries are a convenient and portable snack option. They have a longer shelf life than fresh strawberries and can be enjoyed on their own or added to various dishes and recipes.

6. Versatility:

- Dried strawberries can be used in a wide range of culinary applications. They can be added to cereals, yogurt, granola, trail mix, baked goods (like muffins and cookies), and salads for a burst of flavour and natural sweetness.

7. Lower Water Content:

- The drying process removes the water content from strawberries, concentrating their flavours and nutrients. This also makes dried strawberries less perishable compared to fresh ones.

8. Potential Health Benefits:

- Dried strawberries, like fresh strawberries, are associated with potential health benefits. They may support heart health, aid in weight management due to their fiber content, and provide essential nutrients.

9. Natural Sweetener:

- Dried strawberries can serve as a natural sweetener in recipes. You can chop or grind them into a powder to use as a sweetening agent in smoothies, sauces, and desserts.

10. Snacking and Dessert Component: - Dried strawberries are a popular component in various snack mixes, and they can add a delightful touch to desserts like ice cream and chocolate-covered strawberries.

11. Source of Flavonoids: - Dried strawberries contain flavonoids, which are beneficial compounds that may have various health-promoting properties, including anti-inflammatory effects.

12. Limited Availability: - While fresh strawberries are readily available during their growing season, dried strawberries can be enjoyed year-round, providing access to strawberry flavour even when the fruit is out of season.

13. Potential Sugar Content: - Some commercially available dried strawberries may be sweetened with added sugar or syrup. If you're concerned about added sugars, check the product label for ingredients.

It's important to consume dried strawberries in moderation, as they are calorie-dense due to their concentrated sugars. Additionally, be mindful of any added sugars when purchasing commercial dried strawberries. For the healthiest option, you can also make your own dried strawberries at home without added sugar.

DRIED RASPBERRY TEA

Dried raspberry tea is a delightful herbal infusion made from dried raspberry leaves or dried raspberries. It has a pleasant, slightly fruity and earthy flavour with a hint of sweetness. Raspberry tea is known for its potential health benefits, including being a source of antioxidants and a remedy for various minor ailments. Here's a simple recipe to make dried raspberry tea:

Ingredients:

- 1 to 2 teaspoons of dried raspberry leaves or dried raspberries
- 1 cup of boiling water
- Optional additions: honey, lemon, or other herbs for flavour

Instructions:

- **Prepare the Dried Raspberry Leaves or Raspberries:**
  - If you're using dried raspberry leaves, measure out 1 to 2 teaspoons per cup of tea. If you prefer the flavour of dried raspberries, you can use them in place of the leaves, or use a combination of both.
- **Boil Water:**
  - Bring one cup (8 ounces) of water to a boil in a kettle or on the stovetop.
- **Place the Dried Raspberry Leaves or Raspberries in a Cup:**
  - Put the dried raspberry leaves or raspberries into a teacup or teapot.
- **Pour Boiling Water:**
  - Carefully pour the boiling water over the dried raspberry leaves or raspberries, ensuring they are fully submerged.
- **Steep:**
  - Allow the dried raspberry leaves or raspberries to steep in the hot water for about 5-7 minutes. Adjust the steeping time to your taste, but avoid over-steeping, as it can make the tea overly strong or slightly bitter.
- **Optional Additions:**
  - If desired, you can sweeten your raspberry tea with honey or add a squeeze of lemon for extra flavour.

> Raspberry tea has a naturally pleasant taste, and these additions can enhance it further.

- **Strain (Optional):**
    - If you prefer not to have raspberry leaves or raspberry bits in your tea, use a fine-mesh strainer to remove them while pouring the tea into your cup.
- **Enjoy:**
    - Your dried raspberry tea is now ready to enjoy. Sip it while it's still warm.

Note: Raspberry tea is generally considered safe for most people. However, if you have specific allergies or are pregnant, it's advisable to consult with a healthcare professional before consuming it regularly. Raspberry tea is known for its potential to support women's health and ease discomfort associated with menstruation, but its use should be discussed with a healthcare provider if you have specific health concerns.

Dried raspberries, which are made by removing the moisture from fresh raspberries, offer a unique combination of flavour, nutrients, and convenience. Here are some of the properties and characteristics of dried raspberries:

1. Intense Raspberry Flavour:

- Dried raspberries have a concentrated raspberry flavour that is sweet, slightly tart, and fruity. The drying process intensifies the natural sweetness of the fruit.

2. Nutrient Retention:

- Drying raspberries preserves many of the vitamins and minerals found in fresh raspberries, including vitamin C, manganese, and dietary fiber.

3. Antioxidant Content:

- Dried raspberries, like fresh raspberries, are rich in antioxidants, including anthocyanins and quercetin. Antioxidants help combat oxidative stress and protect cells from damage caused by free radicals.

4. Dietary Fiber:

- Dried raspberries are a source of dietary fiber, which supports digestion, helps maintain regular bowel movements, and may contribute to a feeling of fullness.

5. Convenience:

- Dried raspberries are a convenient and portable snack option. They have a longer shelf life than fresh raspberries and can be enjoyed on their own or added to various dishes and recipes.

6. Versatility:

- Dried raspberries can be used in a wide range of culinary applications. They can be added to cereals, yogurt, oatmeal, granola, trail mix, baked goods (like muffins and cookies), and salads for a burst of raspberry flavour and natural sweetness.

7. Natural Sweetener:

- Dried raspberries can serve as a natural sweetening agent in recipes. You can chop or grind them into a powder to use as a sweetener in smoothies, sauces, and desserts.

8. Limited Availability:

- While fresh raspberries are readily available during their growing season, dried raspberries can be enjoyed year-round, providing access to raspberry flavour even when fresh berries are out of season.

9. Potential Health Benefits:

- Dried raspberries, like fresh raspberries, are associated with potential health benefits. They may support heart health, aid in weight management due to their fiber content, and provide essential nutrients.

10. Source of Flavonoids: - Dried raspberries contain flavonoids, which are beneficial compounds that may have various health-promoting properties, including anti-inflammatory effects.

11. Snacking and Dessert Component: - Dried raspberries are a popular component in various snack mixes, and they can add a delightful touch to desserts like ice cream, yogurt, and chocolate treats.

12. Potential Sugar Content: - Some commercially available dried raspberries may be sweetened with added sugar or syrup. If you're concerned about added sugars, check the product label for ingredients.

It's important to consume dried raspberries in moderation, as they are calorie-dense due to their concentrated sugars. Additionally, be mindful of any added sugars when purchasing commercial dried raspberries. For the healthiest option, you can also make your own dried raspberries at home without added sugar.

Now, let'S mix more ingredients and flavours:

CINNAMON AND ORANGE TEA:

- 1 cinnamon stick
- 1 orange peel (or a few slices of fresh orange)
- 1-2 black tea bags or 1-2 tablespoons loose black tea
- 2 cups of water
- Honey or sugar to taste (optional)

Instructions:

- In a saucepan, combine water, cinnamon, and orange peel.
- Bring to a boil, then reduce heat and simmer for 10-15 minutes.
- Add the tea bags or loose tea and let steep for 3-5 minutes.
- Strain the tea into cups, and sweeten with honey or sugar if desired.

These winter herb tea recipes should provide you with comforting and delicious options to enjoy during the colder months. Feel free to adjust the ingredients and sweetness levels to suit your taste preferences. Stay warm and cozy!

Cinnamon sticks, derived from the bark of cinnamon trees, are a popular spice known for their warm and sweet flavour. They are used in various culinary dishes, beverages, and even for medicinal purposes. Cinnamon sticks have several properties, including:

1. Flavourful and Aromatic:

- Cinnamon sticks impart a sweet, warm, and woody flavour to dishes and beverages. Their aroma is rich and inviting, making them a popular spice in many cuisines.

2. Antioxidant Properties:

- Cinnamon contains antioxidants, such as polyphenols, which can help protect the body's cells from oxidative damage caused by free radicals. These antioxidants may have health benefits.

3. Anti-Inflammatory Effects:

- Cinnamon has anti-inflammatory properties, which may help reduce inflammation in the body. This property is often attributed to compounds like cinnamaldehyde.

4. Potential Blood Sugar Regulation:

- Some studies suggest that cinnamon may help regulate blood sugar levels by improving insulin sensitivity. It may be beneficial for individuals with diabetes or those at risk of developing it.

5. Antibacterial and Antifungal:

- Cinnamon has natural antimicrobial properties. It may help inhibit the growth of bacteria and fungi, making it useful for food preservation and potentially supporting oral health.

6. Possible Cardiovascular Benefits:

- Research has indicated that cinnamon may have a positive impact on heart health. It may help lower blood pressure and cholesterol levels, which are risk factors for heart disease.

7. Anti-Clotting Effects:

- Cinnamon may have mild anti-clotting effects, which could potentially reduce the risk of blood clot formation.

8. Gastrointestinal Soothing:

- Cinnamon is known to have a soothing effect on the digestive system. It may help relieve indigestion, gas, and bloating.

9. Aiding in Weight Management:

- Some people believe that cinnamon can help with weight management by stabilizing blood sugar levels and reducing sugar cravings.

10. Aromatherapy and Relaxation: - The pleasant scent of cinnamon is often used in aromatherapy to promote relaxation and a sense of well-being.

11. Culinary Use: - Cinnamon sticks are used in both sweet and savoury dishes. They can be added to curries, stews, desserts, and beverages like mulled wine or spiced cider.

12. Decorative Uses: - Cinnamon sticks are sometimes used decoratively in crafts, potpourri, and home decorations due to their pleasant aroma and rustic appearance.

It's important to note that while cinnamon has many potential health benefits, it should be consumed in moderation as part of a balanced diet. Some people may also be allergic to cinnamon, so it's advisable to be cautious if you are trying it for the first time. If you have specific health concerns or conditions, consult with a healthcare professional before incorporating large quantities of cinnamon into your diet for therapeutic purposes.

BLACK TEA

Black tea is a type of tea that is more oxidized than green, white, and oolong teas, and it is known for its robust flavour and strong aroma. It is produced from the leaves of the Camellia sinensis plant and has several properties:

1. Caffeine Content:

- Black tea contains caffeine, which is a natural stimulant. A typical cup of black tea has less caffeine than coffee but more than green or white tea. The caffeine content can vary depending on the specific type and brewing time.

2. Antioxidant Properties:

- Black tea is rich in antioxidants, particularly flavonoids, which help combat free radicals in the body. These antioxidants may contribute to various health benefits, including reduced risk of chronic diseases.

3. Heart Health:

- Some research suggests that regular consumption of black tea may support heart health by improving cholesterol levels and reducing the risk of cardiovascular diseases.

4. Improved Digestion:

- Black tea is known to have mild digestive properties. It can help soothe an upset stomach, alleviate nausea, and promote healthy digestion.

5. Energy and Alertness:

- The caffeine in black tea can provide a moderate boost in energy and mental alertness. It's often consumed to help combat fatigue and increase focus.

6. Mental Clarity and Cognitive Function:

- Some studies have indicated that the combination of caffeine and L-theanine found in black tea may enhance cognitive function, including memory and attention.

7. Oral Health:

- Black tea contains compounds that can inhibit the growth of harmful bacteria in the mouth, potentially reducing the risk of dental issues such as cavities and gum disease.

8. Immune Support:

- The antioxidants in black tea may support the immune system by helping to protect against infections and illnesses.

9. Anticancer Properties:

- Some research has suggested that the antioxidants in black tea may have anticancer properties, although more studies are needed in this area.

10. Weight Management: - Black tea may aid in weight management by increasing metabolism and promoting fat oxidation. It is often included in weight loss and diet plans.

11. Stress Reduction: - The act of brewing and sipping a cup of black tea can be calming and may help reduce stress and anxiety.

12. Rich Flavour and Aroma: - Black tea is known for its bold, full-bodied flavour and aromatic qualities. It comes in various regional varieties with distinct taste profiles.

13. Versatility in Culinary Use: - Black tea is used in a wide range of culinary applications, from traditional tea preparation to flavouring desserts, marinades, and sauces.

It's important to note that the health benefits of black tea may vary depending on factors such as the quality of the tea, brewing method, and individual preferences. As with any food or beverage, moderation is key, especially for individuals sensitive to caffeine or with certain medical conditions. If you have specific health concerns or questions about incorporating black tea into your diet, consult with a healthcare professional.

HONEY:

Honey is a natural sweet substance produced by honeybees from the nectar of flowers. It has been consumed by humans for thousands of years and is valued not only for its sweet taste but also for its numerous health and nutritional properties. Here are some of the key properties of honey:

1. Natural Sweetener:

- Honey is a natural and unprocessed sweetener, making it a healthier alternative to refined sugar in many recipes and beverages.

2. Rich in Nutrients:

- Honey contains a variety of vitamins, minerals, and antioxidants, although the exact composition can vary depending on the type of flowers the bees collect nectar from. Common nutrients found in honey include vitamin C, calcium, iron, and potassium.

3. Antioxidant Properties:

- Honey is rich in antioxidants, which can help combat free radicals in the body. Antioxidants in honey may contribute to overall health and potentially reduce the risk of chronic diseases.

4. Antibacterial and Antimicrobial:

- Honey has natural antibacterial and antimicrobial properties. It contains hydrogen peroxide, which can help inhibit the growth of harmful bacteria. This property has made honey a traditional remedy for wound care.

5. Wound Healing:

- Honey has been used for centuries as a topical treatment for wounds, burns, and ulcers. It promotes healing by keeping the wound area moist and preventing infection.

6. Cough and Sore Throat Relief:

- Honey can be soothing for a sore throat and may help reduce coughing, making it a common ingredient in homemade cough remedies. It is often combined with warm water and lemon.

7. Digestive Health:

- Honey can have a soothing effect on the digestive system. It is sometimes used to alleviate symptoms of indigestion or as a natural remedy for constipation.

8. Energy Source:

- Honey is a source of natural energy due to its carbohydrate content, primarily in the form of fructose and glucose. It can provide a quick energy boost when consumed.

9. Allergy Relief (Local Honey):

- Some people believe that consuming local honey may help alleviate seasonal allergies because it can contain trace amounts of pollen from local plants. However, scientific evidence supporting this is limited.

10. Skin Care: - Honey is used in various skincare products for its moisturizing and anti-inflammatory properties. It can be applied as a mask for softening and rejuvenating the skin.

11. Long Shelf Life: - Honey has a remarkably long shelf life and does not spoil. Archaeologists have found pots of honey in ancient Egyptian tombs that are thousands of years old and still perfectly edible.

12. Culinary Versatility: - Honey is a versatile ingredient in cooking and baking, adding sweetness and depth of flavour to a wide range of dishes, from dressings and marinades to desserts and pastries.

While honey offers several health benefits, it is important to consume it in moderation, as it is high in natural sugars and calories. Additionally, infants under one year old should not be given honey due to the risk of infant botulism. Raw honey, in particular, should not be given to infants.

There are several alternatives to sweeten herbal tea if you prefer not to use honey, sugar, or other traditional sweeteners. These alternatives can add sweetness with various flavour profiles and health benefits. Here are some natural sweeteners for herbal tea:

1. Stevia:

- Stevia is a plant-based sweetener that is much sweeter than sugar, so a little goes a long way. It is calorie-free and does not raise blood sugar levels, making it suitable for people with diabetes.

2. Agave Nectar:

- Agave nectar is derived from the agave plant and has a mild, neutral flavour. It is slightly thinner than honey and can be used to sweeten herbal tea. Keep in mind that it's still a source of calories and should be used in moderation.

3. Maple Syrup:

- Pure maple syrup can be used to sweeten herbal tea, providing a rich and earthy sweetness. Choose 100% pure maple syrup without added sugars or artificial flavours.

4. Date Syrup:

- Date syrup is made from dates and has a sweet, caramel-like flavour. It's a natural sweetener with a lower glycemic index compared to sugar, making it a better choice for some individuals.

5. Coconut Sugar:

- Coconut sugar is made from the sap of coconut palm trees. It has a slightly caramel flavour and can be used as a sweetener in herbal tea. It's lower on the glycemic index than regular sugar.

6. Monk Fruit Extract:

- Monk fruit extract is derived from the monk fruit and is a calorie-free sweetener. It can be used in small amounts to sweeten herbal tea without impacting blood sugar levels.

7. Fruit Purees or Juice:

- You can add natural sweetness to your herbal tea by using fruit purees or juice. For example, a splash of unsweetened apple or pear juice can add a fruity sweetness.

8. Cinnamon or Vanilla:

- Enhance the flavour of your herbal tea with the natural sweetness of spices like cinnamon or a drop of pure vanilla extract. These options add depth and aroma to your beverage.

9. Citrus Zest:

- Citrus zest from oranges, lemons, or limes can provide a natural burst of flavour and a touch of sweetness to your herbal tea.

10. Licorice Root: - Licorice root is a natural sweetener often used in herbal teas. It has a naturally sweet taste and can be added to herbal tea blends.

Remember that sweetness preferences vary from person to person, so you may need to experiment to find the sweetener and amount that suits your taste. Additionally, be mindful of any dietary restrictions or health considerations when choosing a sweetener. Always check the labels on store-bought sweeteners to ensure they are free from additives or undesirable ingredients.

Orange peels, the outermost layer of the orange fruit, are often discarded, but they are rich in nutrients and can be used for various purposes. Here are some properties and benefits of orange peels:

1. Nutrient-Rich:

- Orange peels are a good source of vitamins and minerals, including vitamin C, vitamin A, vitamin B6, calcium, potassium, and dietary fiber.

2. Antioxidant Properties:

- Orange peels contain flavonoids and phytonutrients that have antioxidant properties. Antioxidants help protect cells from damage caused by free radicals and may contribute to overall health.

3. Digestive Aid:

- The dietary fiber in orange peels can aid digestion by promoting regular bowel movements and preventing constipation.

4. Weight Management:

- The fiber in orange peels can help you feel full and satisfied, potentially reducing overeating and supporting weight management efforts.

5. Oral Health:

- The natural oils in orange peels have antimicrobial properties and can help freshen breath. Chewing on orange peel or using it as an ingredient in homemade toothpaste may promote oral health.

6. Skin Benefits:

- Orange peel can be used as an ingredient in homemade skincare products due to its natural exfoliating and skin-brightening properties. It can help remove dead skin cells and reduce the appearance of blemishes and dark spots.

7. Aromatherapy:

- The essential oil extracted from orange peels is used in aromatherapy for its uplifting and mood-enhancing properties. It is believed to reduce stress and anxiety.

8. Culinary Uses:

- Dried and powdered orange peel, known as orange zest, is a common culinary ingredient. It is used to add flavour to a wide range of dishes, including desserts, marinades, and sauces.

9. Household Cleaner:

- The natural oils in orange peels can be used to make homemade, eco-friendly cleaning products. They can help cut through grease and leave a pleasant citrus scent.

10. Potpourri and Air Fresheners: - Dried orange peels can be used in potpourri and homemade air fresheners to add a pleasant and refreshing fragrance to your home.

11. Pest Repellent: - The scent of orange peels can deter certain pests like ants and flies. Placing orange peels near entry points or areas where pests are a problem may help keep them away.

12. Reduced Waste: - Using orange peels in various ways can help reduce kitchen waste and promote sustainability.

When using orange peels, it's essential to ensure they are thoroughly washed and free from pesticides or contaminants. Organic oranges may be a preferable choice if you plan to use the peels for culinary or skincare purposes. Additionally, consider the source of your orange peels if you intend to use them for any applications involving ingestion or skin contact.

GINGER, HONEY AND LEMON TEA:

- 1-inch piece of fresh ginger, sliced
- 1 lemon, sliced
- 1-2 tablespoons of honey
- 2 cups of boiling water

Instructions:

- Place the ginger and lemon slices in a teapot or a heatproof pitcher.
- Pour boiling water over the ginger and lemon.
- Let steep for 5-10 minutes.
- Stir in honey to taste.

Fresh ginger, scientifically known as Zingiber officinale, is a popular spice and herbal remedy with a wide range of properties and health benefits. Here are some of the key properties and characteristics of fresh ginger:

1. Anti-Inflammatory:

- Ginger contains bioactive compounds like gingerol, which have potent anti-inflammatory effects. It can help reduce inflammation in the body, potentially alleviating conditions like arthritis.

2. Antioxidant-Rich:

- Ginger is a rich source of antioxidants that help combat oxidative stress and protect cells from damage caused by free radicals.

3. Gastrointestinal Health:

- Ginger has a long history of use in traditional medicine for digestive complaints. It can help relieve nausea, indigestion, and motion sickness. Ginger tea or ginger candies are often used for these purposes.

4. Immune Support:

- Ginger's immune-boosting properties may help the body fight off infections. It is often consumed in tea or incorporated into dishes during the cold and flu season.

5. Pain Relief:

- Ginger may provide pain relief, particularly for menstrual pain and muscle soreness. It may have a mild analgesic effect.

6. Anti-Nausea:

- Ginger is known for its anti-nausea properties and is commonly used to alleviate nausea caused by pregnancy, chemotherapy, or motion sickness. It is often recommended as a natural remedy for morning sickness.

7. Cardiovascular Health:

- Some research suggests that ginger may help lower blood pressure and reduce the risk of heart disease by improving cholesterol levels and reducing triglycerides.

8. Blood Sugar Regulation:

- Ginger may help regulate blood sugar levels and improve insulin sensitivity, potentially benefiting individuals with diabetes or those at risk of developing it.

9. Anti-Cancer Potential:

- Preliminary studies have indicated that ginger may have anticancer properties, potentially inhibiting the growth of cancer cells. However, more research is needed in this area.

10. Anti-Microbial: - Ginger has natural antimicrobial properties and may help inhibit the growth of certain bacteria and fungi.

11. Pain and Inflammation in Osteoarthritis: - Some studies suggest that ginger supplementation may reduce pain and improve joint function in individuals with osteoarthritis.

12. Respiratory Health: - Ginger's anti-inflammatory and antimicrobial properties may help alleviate symptoms of respiratory conditions, such as sore throat or congestion.

13. Culinary Uses: - Fresh ginger is a versatile ingredient in cooking and baking, adding a spicy and aromatic flavour to a wide range of dishes, from stir-fries to soups to desserts.

14. Aromatherapy: - The aroma of fresh ginger is often used in aromatherapy for its stimulating and invigorating effects. It can help improve focus and mental clarity.

It's important to note that while fresh ginger offers many potential health benefits, individual responses can vary. People with certain medical conditions or taking specific medications should consult with a healthcare professional before adding large quantities of ginger to their diet or using it for therapeutic purposes. Additionally, ginger should be consumed in moderation, as excessive intake can lead to digestive discomfort in some individuals.

Fresh lemons, scientifically known as Citrus limon, are a widely consumed citrus fruit known for their vibrant flavour and numerous health properties. Here are some key properties and characteristics of fresh lemons:

1. Rich in Vitamin C:

- Lemons are an excellent source of vitamin C, a powerful antioxidant that supports the immune system, promotes healthy skin, and aids in wound healing.

2. Antioxidant Properties:

- In addition to vitamin C, lemons contain other antioxidants like flavonoids and carotenoids, which help protect cells from oxidative damage caused by free radicals.

3. Alkalizing Effect:

- Despite their acidic taste, lemons have an alkalizing effect on the body when metabolized. This can help balance the body's pH levels.

4. Digestive Health:

- Lemon juice can stimulate the production of digestive enzymes and promote healthy digestion. It is often consumed with warm water in the morning as a natural digestive aid.

5. Detoxification:

- Lemon water is believed to support the body's natural detoxification processes by promoting the production of bile and flushing toxins from the liver and kidneys.

6. Hydration:

- Adding lemon to water can enhance its flavour and encourage increased water intake, helping to keep the body hydrated.

7. Immune Support:

- The vitamin C in lemons is known for its immune-boosting properties. It may help reduce the severity and duration of colds and infections.

8. Skin Health:

- Lemon juice is often used topically to lighten dark spots and blemishes and improve overall skin tone. It may also help reduce excess oil production.

9. Weight Management:

- The fiber in lemons can help increase feelings of fullness and support weight management by reducing overeating.

10. Blood Pressure: - Some studies suggest that the potassium content in lemons may help regulate blood pressure.

11. Antimicrobial Properties: - Lemon juice and lemon zest have natural antimicrobial properties that can help inhibit the growth of certain bacteria and fungi.

12. Anti-Inflammatory Effects: - Lemon contains compounds that may have anti-inflammatory effects, potentially reducing inflammation in the body.

13. Cardiovascular Health: - The antioxidants in lemons may contribute to heart health by reducing the risk of heart disease and improving cholesterol levels.

14. Alleviation of Kidney Stones: - Lemon juice may help prevent the formation of kidney stones by increasing citrate levels in the urine.

15. Aromatherapy: - The refreshing and invigorating scent of lemon essential oil is used in aromatherapy to improve mood, reduce stress, and increase mental clarity.

16. Culinary Uses: - Lemons are a versatile ingredient in cooking and baking, adding a tangy and citrusy flavour to a wide range of dishes, from salads to marinades to desserts.

It's important to note that while lemons offer many potential health benefits, their high acidity can be harsh on tooth enamel. To minimize this effect, it's advisable to consume lemon juice diluted in water and avoid brushing your teeth immediately after consumption. Additionally, individuals with citrus allergies or sensitivities should exercise caution when consuming lemons.

PEPPERMINT MOCHA HERBAL TEA:

- 1 peppermint tea bag
- 1 cocoa powder or cacao powder
- 1 cup of boiling water
- 1-2 tablespoons of honey or sweetener of your choice (optional)
- Whipped cream for topping (optional)

Instructions:

- Place the peppermint tea bag and cocoa powder in a cup.
- Pour boiling water over the tea bag and let it steep for 3-5 minutes.
- Remove the tea bag and stir in honey or sweetener if desired.
- Top with whipped cream for an extra treat.

Dried peppermint, also known as dried mint, is a popular herb with a wide range of properties and uses. It is derived from the leaves of the peppermint plant (Mentha × piperita) and is known for its refreshing aroma and flavour. Here are some of the key properties and characteristics of dried peppermint:

1. Aromatic and Flavourful:

- Dried peppermint leaves have a strong and refreshing minty aroma and flavour. They are commonly used to add a cooling and invigorating taste to various dishes and beverages.

2. Digestive Aid:

- Peppermint is well-known for its digestive properties. Consuming dried peppermint tea or adding it to meals may help alleviate indigestion, bloating, and gas. It can also promote the flow of bile, aiding in digestion.

3. Soothing Properties:

- Peppermint is often used to soothe upset stomachs and relieve nausea. It can be beneficial for those experiencing motion sickness or morning sickness during pregnancy.

4. Antispasmodic Effects:

- Dried peppermint has antispasmodic properties that may help relax the muscles of the gastrointestinal tract, making it useful for managing irritable bowel syndrome (IBS) symptoms and cramps.

5. Respiratory Health:

- Peppermint's menthol content can help open airways and provide relief from congestion and respiratory discomfort when consumed as a tea or inhaled through steam.

6. Mental Alertness:

- The aroma of peppermint is invigorating and can help improve mental clarity and concentration. It is often used in aromatherapy for this purpose.

7. Antioxidant Properties:

- Peppermint contains antioxidants that help protect cells from oxidative stress and may contribute to overall health.

8. Pain Relief:

- Topical peppermint oil or peppermint-infused creams may provide relief from headaches, muscle pain, and joint pain when applied to the affected area.

9. Allergy Relief:

- Peppermint may help alleviate allergy symptoms, such as a runny nose or itchy eyes, due to its anti-inflammatory and antihistamine-like properties.

10. Antimicrobial and Antibacterial: - Peppermint has natural antimicrobial and antibacterial properties that can help inhibit the growth of certain bacteria and fungi.

11. Culinary Uses: - Dried peppermint is a common ingredient in culinary dishes, including salads, desserts, and beverages like herbal teas and mojitos.

12. Skin Care: - Peppermint can be used topically in skincare products for its cooling and soothing effects. It may help reduce skin irritation and redness.

13. Relaxation: - Peppermint tea can have a calming effect, making it a popular choice for relaxation and stress relief.

14. Potential Weight Management: - Some people find that peppermint tea helps curb appetite and reduce cravings, potentially aiding in weight management efforts.

15. Long Shelf Life: - Dried peppermint has a long shelf life and can be stored for an extended period without losing its flavour or aroma.

Dried peppermint can be used in various forms, including loose leaves, tea bags, and as an ingredient in spice blends and herbal remedies. It is generally well-tolerated, but some individuals may be sensitive to mint and should use it in moderation. Additionally, it's important to consult with a healthcare professional before using peppermint or its extracts for therapeutic purposes, especially if you have specific medical conditions or are taking medications.

Cocoa powder is derived from the cacao bean and is used primarily as a key ingredient in chocolate products and various recipes. It is available in both natural (unsweetened) and Dutch-processed (alkalized) varieties, each with its unique properties. Here are some of the key properties and characteristics of cocoa powder:

1. Flavour and Aroma:

- Cocoa powder has a rich and deep chocolate flavour with aromatic notes. Its flavour can range from mildly bitter to intensely chocolatey, depending on the type and processing method.

2. Antioxidant-Rich:

- Cocoa powder is a potent source of antioxidants, particularly flavonoids, which can help combat oxidative stress and inflammation. These antioxidants are associated with potential health benefits.

3. Mood Enhancement:

- Cocoa contains compounds like theobromine and phenylethylamine, which can have mood-enhancing effects. They may contribute to feelings of well-being and pleasure.

4. Cardiovascular Health:

- Some studies suggest that the antioxidants in cocoa may have cardiovascular benefits, including reducing blood pressure and improving cholesterol levels. This is often attributed to flavonoids like epicatechin.

5. Brain Health:

- The consumption of cocoa and its flavonoids has been linked to improved cognitive function and may offer neuroprotective benefits.

6. Skin Health:

- Cocoa polyphenols have been studied for their potential to protect the skin against UV radiation and improve skin elasticity. Cocoa-based skincare products are popular for these reasons.

7. Natural Sweetness:

- Cocoa powder itself is not very sweet, but it can provide a natural chocolate flavour to recipes without the need for excessive added sugar.

8. Culinary Versatility:

- Cocoa powder is a versatile ingredient used in a wide range of sweet and savoury recipes. It is commonly used in baking, hot chocolate, chocolate sauces, smoothies, and desserts.

9. High in Minerals:

- Cocoa powder is a good source of essential minerals, including magnesium, iron, calcium, and potassium. These minerals play important roles in various bodily functions.

10. Weight Management: - Cocoa powder, especially the unsweetened variety, can be used as a lower-calorie substitute for chocolate in recipes, making it suitable for those who are conscious of calorie intake.

11. Natural Coloring: - Cocoa powder is used in food production for its natural brown color. It can be used to color and flavour various food items, including chocolate, ice cream, and baked goods.

12. Limited Fat Content: - Unsweetened cocoa powder is relatively low in fat, making it a good choice for those looking to reduce fat intake.

13. Caffeine Content: - Cocoa naturally contains caffeine, though the amount is relatively low compared to coffee or tea. It can provide a mild energy boost.

14. Varieties: - There are different types of cocoa powder, including natural (non-alkalized) and Dutch-processed (alkalized). Dutch-processed cocoa is less acidic and has a milder flavour, making it preferred for recipes where a less intense chocolate flavour is desired.

It's important to note that while cocoa powder offers potential health benefits, many commercial chocolate products and recipes containing cocoa may also include added sugars and fats, which can affect the overall nutritional profile. When incorporating cocoa powder into your diet, consider the full ingredient list and portion sizes to make healthier choices. Additionally, individuals with certain medical conditions, such as chocolate allergies or caffeine sensitivities, should exercise caution when consuming cocoa products.

Cocoa powder and **cacao powder** are both derived from the cacao bean, but they undergo different processing methods, which result in distinct flavour profiles and nutritional properties. Here are the main differences between cocoa powder and cacao powder:

1. Processing:

- **Cocoa Powder:** Cocoa powder is produced by roasting cacao beans at high temperatures, which can reduce some of the natural bitterness and acidity of the cacao. It is then ground into a fine powder. Most commercial cocoa powders are also processed with alkali (Dutch-processed) to further reduce acidity and bitterness.
- **Cacao Powder:** Cacao powder is made by cold-pressing unroasted cacao beans. This process preserves more of the cacao's natural enzymes and nutrients, resulting in a purer and less processed product. Cacao powder is typically considered less processed than cocoa powder.

2. Flavour:

- **Cocoa Powder:** Cocoa powder, especially Dutch-processed cocoa, tends to have a milder and less bitter flavour compared to cacao powder. It has a classic chocolate flavour and is commonly used in baking and making hot cocoa.
- **Cacao Powder:** Cacao powder has a more intense and pronounced chocolate flavour. It often retains the natural fruity and slightly bitter notes of the cacao bean, giving it a richer and more complex taste.

3. Nutritional Content:

- **Cocoa Powder:** Due to the high-temperature roasting and additional processing, cocoa powder may have slightly fewer antioxidants and nutrients than cacao powder. However, it is still a good source of minerals like iron, calcium, and potassium.
- **Cacao Powder:** Cacao powder is considered more nutritionally dense because it undergoes minimal processing. It is rich in antioxidants, particularly flavonoids, and contains higher levels of minerals and vitamins, such as magnesium, iron, and vitamin C.

4. Uses:

- **Cocoa Powder:** Cocoa powder is commonly used in baking, making chocolate-flavoured desserts, and preparing hot chocolate. It is often the preferred choice for recipes that require a milder chocolate flavour.
- **Cacao Powder:** Cacao powder is often used in recipes where a more intense chocolate flavour is desired. It is popular in making raw chocolate, smoothie bowls, energy bars, and other health-conscious recipes. It is also used in some traditional Mesoamerican and South American dishes.

5. Health Considerations:

- **Cocoa Powder:** Cocoa powder is still a relatively healthy option and offers some health benefits due to its antioxidant content. However, it may not be as nutrient-dense as cacao powder.
- **Cacao Powder:** Cacao powder is often considered the healthier choice due to its higher nutrient content and minimal processing. It is particularly valued for its antioxidant properties and potential health benefits.

In summary, the main difference between cocoa powder and cacao powder lies in the processing methods and resulting flavour and nutrient profiles. Cocoa powder is more commonly found in everyday baking and chocolate products, while cacao powder is favored in health-conscious recipes and those seeking a more intense chocolate flavour with potential health benefits. When choosing between the two, consider the specific needs of your recipe and your preference for flavour and nutrition.

SPICED CHAI TEA:

- 1 cinnamon stick
- 4-5 whole cloves
- 4-5 cardamom pods
- 1-inch piece of fresh ginger, sliced
- 1-2 black tea bags or 1-2 tablespoons loose black tea
- 2 cups of water
- 1 cup of milk (dairy or non-dairy)
- Honey or sugar to taste (optional)

Instructions:

- In a saucepan, combine water, spices, and ginger. Bring to a boil, then reduce heat and simmer for 10-15 minutes.
- Add the tea bags or loose tea and let steep for 3-5 minutes.
- Add the milk and heat until hot but not boiling.
- Strain the tea into cups and sweeten with honey or sugar if desired.

Whole cloves are a spice derived from the dried flower buds of the clove tree (Syzygium aromaticum). They are a popular spice in many cuisines and have a strong, warm, and sweet flavour with a hint of bitterness. Cloves are used in both sweet and savoury dishes and are also valued for their potential medicinal properties. Here are some of the properties and characteristics of whole cloves:

1. Flavourful Spice:

- Cloves have a distinctive and intense flavour. They are known for their warm, sweet, and slightly peppery taste, which adds depth and complexity to dishes.

2. Aromatic:

- Whole cloves have a strong and pleasing aroma characterized by their sweet and spicy scent. They are often used in potpourri and other aromatic preparations.

3. Culinary Uses:

- Cloves are a versatile spice used in various culinary applications, including spice blends, curries, stews, pickles, and baked goods like gingerbread and fruitcakes.

4. Toothache Relief:

- Cloves have been traditionally used for their potential analgesic properties. Eugenol, a compound found in cloves, can act as a natural anesthetic and may help alleviate toothache pain. Clove oil is often used for this purpose.

5. Potential Antioxidant Properties:

- Cloves are rich in antioxidants, which help protect cells from oxidative stress and free radical damage. Antioxidants in cloves may contribute to overall health.

6. Anti-Inflammatory Effects:

- Eugenol, the primary active compound in cloves, has demonstrated anti-inflammatory properties and may help reduce inflammation and related discomfort.

7. Digestive Aid:

- Cloves have been used to support digestion and relieve digestive discomfort. They may help alleviate symptoms such as gas, bloating, and indigestion.

8. Respiratory Health:

- Clove oil or clove-infused teas are sometimes used to soothe respiratory issues like coughs and bronchitis. The aroma of cloves can also help clear congestion.

9. Potential Antimicrobial Properties:

- Cloves contain compounds with potential antimicrobial properties, which may help combat bacteria, fungi, and parasites. They have been used in traditional medicine for this purpose.

10. Natural Preservative: - Due to their antimicrobial properties, cloves have been used historically as a natural food preservative, particularly in pickling and preserving.

11. Insect Repellent: - Clove oil can be used as a natural insect repellent. It is often added to lotions or applied topically to deter insects like mosquitoes.

12. Potpourri and Fragrance: - Whole cloves are used in potpourri, sachets, and scented candles for their pleasant aroma. They can add a warm and spicy note to fragrance blends.

13. Potential Blood Sugar Regulation: - Some research suggests that cloves may help regulate blood sugar levels, making them potentially beneficial for individuals with diabetes. However, more research is needed to confirm these effects.

It's important to use whole cloves in moderation, as their strong flavour can easily overpower a dish. They are often used whole in recipes but can also be ground into a powder for specific culinary applications. Clove oil is highly concentrated and should be used sparingly and diluted when applied topically or ingested. As with any spice or herbal remedy, individual responses may vary, and it's advisable to consult with a healthcare professional for specific health concerns or treatments involving cloves.

Cardamom pods, also known simply as cardamom, are a popular spice with a unique and aromatic flavour. These small green pods contain tiny black seeds and are used in various culinary and medicinal applications. Here are some properties and characteristics of cardamom pods:

1. Distinctive Flavour:

- Cardamom pods have a complex and distinctive flavour profile. They are known for their sweet, spicy, and slightly citrusy taste with hints of mint and eucalyptus.

2. Versatile Spice:

- Cardamom is a versatile spice used in a wide range of dishes, both sweet and savoury. It is a common ingredient in Indian, Middle Eastern, and Scandinavian cuisines.

3. Two Varieties:

- There are two main varieties of cardamom: green cardamom (Elettaria cardamomum) and black cardamom (Amomum subulatum or Amomum costatum). Green cardamom is the most common and has a milder flavour, while black cardamom has a smoky, earthy flavour and is typically used in savoury dishes.

4. Aromatic Spice:

- Cardamom pods have a strong and pleasant aroma characterized by their sweet and spicy scent. They are often used to flavour desserts, beverages, and various dishes.

5. Culinary Uses:

- Cardamom pods are used in various culinary applications, including curries, rice dishes, biryanis, desserts like ice cream and cakes, and beverages like chai tea and mulled wine.

6. Potential Digestive Aid:

- Cardamom is traditionally used as a digestive aid. It may help relieve symptoms of indigestion, gas, and bloating. Chewing on cardamom pods after a meal is a common practice in some cultures.

7. Antioxidant Content:

- Cardamom is a source of antioxidants, which help protect cells from oxidative stress and free radical damage.

8. Potential Anti-Inflammatory Properties:

- Some studies suggest that cardamom may have anti-inflammatory effects and could help reduce inflammation and related discomfort.

9. Respiratory Health:

- Cardamom is used in traditional medicine to support respiratory health. It may help relieve symptoms of coughs and congestion and clear the airways.

10. Natural Breath Freshener: - Chewing on cardamom pods or consuming cardamom-infused mouth fresheners can help combat bad breath due to its pleasant aroma.

11. Aromatherapy: - Cardamom essential oil, extracted from the seeds, is used in aromatherapy for its potential calming and uplifting effects.

12. Potential Blood Sugar Regulation: - Some research suggests that cardamom may help regulate blood sugar levels and improve insulin sensitivity, making it potentially beneficial for individuals with diabetes. However, more research is needed to confirm these effects.

13. Perfumery and Fragrance: - Cardamom's aromatic qualities make it a popular ingredient in perfumery and fragrance blends.

14. Natural Preservative: - Due to its antimicrobial properties, cardamom has been used historically as a natural food preservative.

Cardamom pods are typically used in cooking by lightly crushing or grinding them to release the seeds, which contain the intense flavour. They can be added whole to rice dishes or used in spice blends. The seeds can also be ground into a powder for more convenient use in recipes. Whether in culinary or medicinal applications, cardamom pods are valued for their unique flavour and potential health benefits.

Any ingredients mentioned in the recipes are easy to buy online. Whether you are an Amazon.com fan or you prefer your local herbal shops, you can get any herbs, dried fruits or a lovely teapot to infuse your tea.

www.ingramcontent.com/pod-product-compliance
Lightning Source LLC
Chambersburg PA
CBHW070819280726
48660CB00016B/2139